SUIC PREVENTION HANDBOOK

A MENTAL HEALTH GUIDE FOR SAVING LIVES

SECOND EDITION

BEN OAKLEY

Twelvetrees Camden, United Kingdom
www.twelvetreescamden.com

SUICIDE PREVENTION HANDBOOK

A MENTAL HEALTH GUIDE FOR SAVING LIVES

by Ben Oakley

SECOND EDITION

Independently Published

ISBN: 9798541916508

Cover design by Marina Luisa & Ben Oakley

Discover more:

www.benoakley.co.uk

"It's only right that we pass on any knowledge we have to others so that it may better benefit their lives."

Ben Oakley.

Suicide Prevention Handbook

A lot of work has gone into publishing this book for you, using real-world psychiatric processes and established mental health guidance. I hope the exercises and guides within can help you to help yourself or another.

CHAPTER LIST

SUICIDE PREVENTION HANDBOOK

SECOND EDITION

This Book Is for You!

This second edition of the Suicide Prevention Handbook is universally aimed at anyone of any age from any walk of life.

This handbook is for YOU, no matter who you are.

This book provides you with the tools and knowledge to save your own life or the life of another. It's easy to read, digest, and navigate with the sole purpose of preventing you or another person taking their own life.

You can become a hero just by reaching out to someone who might be struggling. You can also become a hero by overcoming negative thought and emotion to help yourself. More on being a hero in a moment!

The World Health Organisation (WHO) set out international recommendations for suicide prevention. The report, sent to the leaders of our countries, included four steps.

- Surveillance.
- Identification of risks and protective factors.
- Development & evaluation of interventions.
- Implementation.

Surveillance in terms of suicide prevention means to systematically collect data on suicides and suicide attempts. This book you have in your hands or on your screen is focused on parts two and three of the WHO recommendations.

- Identification of risks and protective factors.
- Development and evaluation of interventions.

To make it even more simple, I've broken that down into a new and more accessible four step plan that anyone can use to gain knowledge and awareness from.

The FOUR-STEP PLAN:

- Warning Signs
- Risk Factors
- Intervention
- Coping Strategies

Each section gives you all the information you need to reach out or seek help yourself. Unlike many other mental health and suicide prevention guides, this book doesn't hold anything back or beat around the bush. This book gets straight to the point.

If you want to know what to say to a person who is struggling then **this book shows you exactly what you can say**.

It doesn't mean you *have* to use it but it's there as an option if it works for you. The section on intervention goes into how to start a conversation, what questions to ask and then how to guide a conversation away from negativity.

The words written here talk directly to you as if we are in the same room having a conversation or presenting to you at a seminar.

This book is written in British English with some American English elements added only when describing an American saying or place name. The book mostly uses UK statistics with some international statistics thrown in for relevancy.

On top of the expansive four-step plan, you'll also find a guide on how to create a suicide prevention life plan. There's also a section where we debunk mental health myths and discuss the social reasons behind the rise of male suicide.

Certain studies cited or quotes used can be found in the extensive bibliography at the back of the book. Included for your benefit is an extensive mental health organisation and helpline list.

Now, let's get back to being a hero!

What does it mean to be a hero?

Being a hero doesn't always mean running into a burning building, rescuing someone's who's trapped inside then jumping off the roof with a rope tied to your waist. You can also save someone who is feeling trapped **right now**.

It doesn't don't mean being physically trapped in a burning building, it's talking about being mentally trapped in a moment of time that has become an entire existence for someone.

The analogy of being trapped in a burning building isn't too far from the truth of mental illness. It does feel like we're trapped in our bodies, unable to climb out from the darkness that has fallen all around us. Someone feeling that way needs rescuing just as much as someone trapped in a burning building.

Why would someone want to be a hero?

- To be known as a hero?
- For their own self-esteem?
- They have a hero complex?
- They desire attention they failed to receive in earlier life?
- It makes them happy to help others?
- Were they once in need of rescue and no-one came for them?
- Have they been pushed into the role of hero?

The correct answer is; it doesn't matter! We can be heroes for the right or wrong reason but if we can reach out and save a life then we can change the world one small step at a time. There's a difference between talking about mental health and actively reaching out.

The UK loses approximately 6,500 people to suicide each year and yet we still don't really acknowledge it as a genuine problem. On average, 5,000 of those deaths are male suicides.

Let's repeat that; an average of 6,500 people are lost to suicide in the UK each and every year. It's surely time that suicide was labelled a pandemic.

It Doesn't Matter

There are more regional accents in the UK than there are anywhere else in the world when comparing the size of geographical areas.

How do you refer to people you are friends with?

- Amigo
- Babe
- Blud
- Bro
- Bruv

- Buddy
- Chum
- Cocker
- Comrade
- Cuz
- Fam
- Fella
- Friend
- Frosty Jim
- Fshizzle My Nizzle
- Geezer
- Hetso
- Honey
- Horsebox
- Lad
- Mate
- Pal

Alright, I threw in the last two to see if you're still paying attention but you get the point.

It doesn't matter how you speak.

It doesn't matter where you come from or what your background is.

It doesn't matter where you live or what class you think you belong to.

It doesn't matter if you don't know who you are right now.

What matters is that your life and the lives of others around you are important. You have it within you to save the life of another. It doesn't matter if they're your mate or your bruv, they're worth saving.

It all sounds rather good doesn't it? Reach out to another, help them through a bad time, save their life, become a hero. It even sounds easy but it's not. It takes dedication and resolve to really save someone. The point here is not to do it for your own glory and benefit but for the benefit of that person and their life.

For when one person takes their own life, they leave multiple others suffering and in pain for quite some time. In fact, many people don't get over the loss of a loved one to suicide and it can even go as far as affecting their own suicidal ideation and life choices.

"I like to use the hard times in the past to motivate me today."

Dwayne Johnson, actor and former wrestler

No One Is Immune

There is no single cause for suicide.

People from all walks of life and all ages can be at risk from suicidal tendencies.

Suicide is generally not an immediate response to emotional instability. It is usually something that has been thought about or planned, it's not normally an opportunistic act. This means that you can still reach those who are at risk. There is still time to save your life or the life of another.

There is **always** time and there is **always** hope.

Now let's get those all-important statistics out of the way. Previously, all four countries that made up the United Kingdom; England, Wales, Scotland, and Northern Ireland, had their data easily accessible but then Coronavirus hit.

The 2019 data is released towards the end of 2020 but is skewed due to coroners being overrun with Coronavirus victims. Northern Ireland are still to release suicide figures for 2019. The following statistics are for 2019, and are the latest available as of Summer 2021, for England, Wales, and Scotland.

Across England, Wales, and Scotland, in 2019, **6,524** suicides were registered by the Office Of National Statistics (ONS).

- 4,923 were male suicides.
- 1,601 were female.

The 2019 figures were an increase from 5,821 total registered suicides (including Northern Ireland), two years earlier, in 2017.

To put it another way; the suicide rate across the country – and world - is increasing, and males make up three out of four suicides in the UK. This has shockingly been the case since the mid-1990s.

When discussing male suicide, we include suicides over the age of 14-years-old. Deaths from an event of '*undetermined intent*' from age 10 to 14-years-old are not included. Although for older teenagers and adults it is assumed that in these deaths the harm was self-inflicted. For younger children it is not clear whether this assumption is appropriate and is therefore not included.

It's not getting better, it's getting worse, but together we can change that.

We must still never forget that suicide is a universal curse and that tens of thousands more take their lives across the world.

In the past decade there has been an increase in suicide of males in their early Twenties, which is worrying. Until 2018, there had been a decrease in overall suicides in the UK since 2013. 2018 bucked the trend by showing an **11.8% increase** from the 2017 figures, and is already higher than that for 2019, without the Northern Ireland figures.

2020's preliminary figures are expected to be higher than all previous years.

2020 could be the worst year for suicides since the mid-1990's and that's down to numerous factors including the Coronavirus pandemic. The Royal College Of Psychiatrists predicted a tsunami of mental health cases after Coronavirus lock-down measures were lifted and they turned out to be right.

We've hit an unprecedented point for mental health in our society.

Mental health awareness is nothing to be ashamed of, it's something that should be embedded into our minds, our society, and culture as early as possible in our lives.

A study by the World Health Organisation (WHO) in 2008, compared methods of suicides between countries and found that the difference is driven primarily by the availability of means.

- Hanging was the most common method in the United Kingdom.
- Firearms were the most common method in the United States.
- Jumping from a tall building was the most common method in Hong Kong.

Males tend to choose a more violent method, such as hanging or suicide by firearm. Whereas females choose less violent methods, such as poisoning.

Now, let's get down to the reason you're here and begin our journey through suicide prevention.

The Warning Signs

There are numerous suicide warning signs to be aware of. Some might seem mundane and irrelevant but that's where knowledge comes into it. If you can understand the warning signs of suicide and deteriorating mental health then you will be better placed to step in.

How many times have you noticed a friend is more distant than usual? What did you do about it?

Mostly, we would just pat them on the back and tell them everything is going to be alright. It helps momentarily but it's not getting to the root cause of the issues they may be going through. If they don't want to talk then you shouldn't just walk away, you should never give up.

You should persevere.

"Each and every one of us make up the threads of human civilisation, just as the roots of a tree reach out for sustenance."

Social Signs

Social signs are those that occur in a social environment or as part of various social interactions such as drinking, drugs, or conversations. They are warning signs that are present in an immediate physical and social setting where people live or where a situation occurs.

Social signs can also be seen in a culture or society that a person is raised into or lives in. Social environment does not differentiate between class, race, or age, it is simply the setting in which a person exists on a social basis.

Alcohol Misuse

This is especially relevant if a person is not usually the type to drink a lot. There's nothing wrong with going out once or twice a week and having drinks with friends. It's how you moderate and approach the amount of drinking that lays out the framework for the evening.

Binge-drinking is a danger and is a common sight in British cities on a Friday or Saturday night. There's nothing wrong with drinking in moderation but there is something unordinary about drinking so much that you end the night passed out or throwing up.

"No sympathy for the devil; keep that in mind. Buy the ticket, take the ride, and if it occasionally gets a little heavier than what you had in mind, well maybe chalk it up to forced consciousness expansion: Tune in, freak out, get beaten."

Hunter S. Thompson, Fear and Loathing in Las Vegas

Heavy drinking can be a way to deal with negative emotions and mask what we perceive as reality. Binge-drinking is the quickest way to disconnect from reality and it has a greater mental health impact on us than most realise. This is especially true of those who seek solace in drinking large amounts of alcohol behind closed doors.

Alcohol is found in the system of more and more people who take their own life. It's vitally important that we can learn to moderate so that we can teach others to moderate.

If your friend offers to buy a drink after having had many drinks before then be the one to decline and say you've had enough. It might seem impossible on a night out when the sole purpose is to get completely drunk but there are ways of getting around it.

The difficulty comes in not knowing what to say, and when you do say something you'll probably get one of the reactions below. It's how you respond to those reactions that make the difference.

Reaction:

"You haven't had that much to drink."

Responses:

"I don't want to lose control of my actions or thoughts."

"I'm happy where I am, no need for more."

"I'm better at drinking than I am at being drunk."

Reaction:

"You're a lightweight."

Responses:

"Then get me my lightweight mug."

"Do you want me passed out or conversational?"

"I don't want any more at the moment, thank you."

Reaction:

"You're so boring."

Responses:

"I'm cutting back for my health and I'd appreciate your help"

"I'm okay with that as long as I'm not completely wasted."

You don't have to be deadly serious with responses to peer pressure and drinking. Making light of a situation can help break down the barrier between you and someone who might need help.

If you know someone is binge-drinking to block out their emotional state then you should really step in. If there's no pressing need to take the drink away from them then use the alcohol to your advantage.

When we consume alcohol, it lowers our emotional defences and sees us becoming more open and confident within social interactions. We can use that to help an individual and it's easier than you might think. It's in no way suggesting to take advantage of someone who is drunk but it might be an opportunity to have them open up about their feelings.

If alcohol drops someone's defences then it would seem like a perfect time to step in and talk to them about how they're feeling and if there's anything you can help with.

Just two questions can change the course of a night or even a life.

(Q) "How are you feeling?"

(Q) "Is there anything I can help with?"

Don't stop there, listen to what they respond with and organically grow into the conversation together. You might see they're on the verge of opening up but are struggling to take that step. That's when you move them to a quieter area to get them talking.

They say that talking therapy is one of the most therapeutic ways to help with ill mental health and it's as true as it has ever been. Just one conversation can lift a huge weight off someone's chest, even if you don't have the answers they're looking for.

Having answers and having a conversation are two completely different things. You won't have the answers to everything and you're far from being alone. Governments don't have the answer to everything, nor do scientists, writers, academics, or scholars. Even religious texts or the Hitchhikers Guide To The Galaxy don't really have the answers to everything.

"Would it save you a lot of time if I just gave up and went mad now?"

Douglas Adams, The Hitchhiker's Guide to the Galaxy

Drug Misuse

In a similar way to alcohol misuse, drug addiction or consuming a large quantity of drugs can be a sign of suicidal ideation. There are those that can seemingly function in high society by shoving as much up their nose as possible. They do it to exist in a social environment they believe accepts them for who they are.

If you're taking drugs to fit in then it's one path to opening up an entire realm of mental health issues. On one hand, it completely takes you out of reality and creates a new world for you to exist in. On the other hand, when those around you stop taking drugs, and you continue, then you're going to feel even worse when you realise that you've become a drug addict by your own hand.

People take drugs for many individual reasons but the most common reason is and always has been to be socially relevant within a circle of peers. From there, some people may become addicted and begin to rely on the reality that drugs are offering. If they are seeking to cloud themselves from their own reality then their addiction will only increase without professional help.

There are clear signs between smoking marijuana and mental health problems in later life, even more so with some Class A drugs. LSD, Cocaine, and Opiates in particular have been linked with various mental health disorders later in life.

Being stoned all day isn't living, it's simply existing in a veil of smoke and paranoia. It's an addiction, in a similar way as smoking tobacco or drinking alcohol can become addictive, though tobacco and alcohol can be more damaging in the long run than marijuana. Addiction can be a cause of mental health problems and it's important to know this when you look at the people around you.

If you know someone who is not usually a drug-taker but is now heavily into drugs then it could be a call for help. Getting them the right help and assistance to wean off drugs is the first thing to do.

We look at how to get help further into this handbook.

Talking About Suicide or Death

It's not common for most people to spark up conversations about suicide, which is why if someone does then you really need to listen.

Any of the following are indicative of someone thinking about suicide and are signs to not just look out for but to **LISTEN** out for.

- Claiming that suicide is the right way to die.
- Talking about suicides they heard on the news.
- Saying it's better to take your own life rather than be killed.

- Saying there is nothing wrong with suicide.
- What will be written on their headstone.
- Who will turn up to their funeral.
- Believing that suicide will make them immortal.
- Seeing suicide as the only way to enter heaven.
- Talking about an endgame which involves their death.
- Wanting to follow in the footsteps of a well-known person who took their own life.
- Talking positively about suicide cults.
- Wanting to create a suicide pact.
- Asking for help in planning a suicide.
- Talking about methods of suicide.
- Talking about where to buy the means or tools with which to take their own life.

Talking about death is slightly different and isn't necessarily focused on suicide. There are some sub-cultures such as the goth crowd or horror fanatics who actively talk about death as part of their lifestyle. Fundamentally there is **nothing wrong with talking about death**, it can actually empower us to know that death will one day come.

The ability to appreciate a knowledge of death can make us live life that little bit better than we might already do. Death in music tastes, horror films, horror books and art is embedded into the lifestyle of how some choose to enjoy life. It's no surprise that self-harm is more prevalent in metal, goth or emo cultures than in others.

It still doesn't make it right.

Just because someone else is doing something doesn't mean that you have to do it. Just because some people talk about death more doesn't mean you shouldn't intervene.

A life is a life, a soul is a soul. Everyone is deserving of life.

You could guide conversations away from suicide and negativity with some of the following:

- "I'd rather talk about life than death."
- "Life is more important than death."
- "Suicide is a permanent solution to a temporary problem."
- "No-one should suffer so badly that they choose to take their own life."
- Ask if they have felt this way before.
- Let them know that you care about them.
- Encourage them to seek professional help.

Then get them talking about their emotions and feelings.

- What's going on in their life?
- Why do they feel this way?
- What can you do to help?

"Caring about mental health doesn't mean pasting statistics on social media, waiting for like and then moving on. It means that you are actively reaching out to others."

Personal Signs

Feeling Of Hopelessness

A lack of hope can open up the mind to negative thoughts and emotions. It can lead to ill mental health and a despondent attitude which can create far more serious issues down the line.

Someone could lose hope for any reason and it might seem mundane to you but it could be life-changing for another.

The following can be signs of losing hope:

- Lack of progression in a career.
- Not finding the right relationship.

- Lack of a future.
- Believing there is nothing better out there.
- Seeing themselves as weak and as a burden.
- Falling into debt.
- Not being able to socialise well with others.
- Feeling that everything they do is wrong.
- Hating their body and the way they think.
- Waking up each day feeling worthless.
- Losing interest in regular activities.
- Not being able to enjoy anything.
- Thinking of themselves as worthless.
- Questioning their entire life.
- Believing they will be stuck in the same life forever.
- Constantly thinking negative or destructive thoughts.

It's usually a **lack of something** that drives people to lose hope.

We need hopes and dreams in our lives because without them we're running on empty. Dreams drive us forward and see us become stronger people. Hopes are the things we hold onto when we're feeling down, they offer us a glimmer of what we are aiming to achieve or grow into.

To lose hope can lead to low self-esteem, lack of confidence and negative emotions.

"There is no greater disease than the loss of hope."

Yisroel Salanter, father of the Musar movement.

Feeling Of Disconnection

Do you know how it feels to not know the world you live in anymore? It's a feeling most people have on a regular basis but it's how you deal with it that makes the difference.

A disconnect from reality can be one of the most upsetting things to ever happen. It's as if anxiety, stress, and withdrawal combine all at once to remove you from the world you know. A greyness falls over the world and a sense of doom and hopelessness becomes your new reality.

The danger is when someone continuously goes down a path of multiple disconnects. When someone loses touch with reality, you might see or hear them do any of the following:

- Stop talking as much.
- Not making much sense when they do talk.

- Being confused about their life.
- A lack of emotion.
- Withdrawal from previously enjoyed activities.
- Uncharacteristic risk-taking.
- Loss of personal hygiene.
- Disinterest in their appearance.
- Not responding to messages.
- Wondering why the world is so painful.

Uncharacteristic risk-taking means to do things they wouldn't normally do. It could be something such as aggressively approaching others or walking out into traffic without a second thought.

It might be different if they decide to do a sky-jump because the risk is minimised by professionals. Yet, if they want to stand on top of tall buildings to see how it feels then you might have a reason to worry.

Previous Suicidal Behaviour

It comes as no surprise to learn that over 30% of people who take their own lives in the UK have either attempted suicide before or had been actively planning it. If you know someone who has previously tried or thought about taking their own life then they are **still in danger** of doing so. It's a thought process that doesn't go away overnight and can take a long time to really get over, if at all.

If someone tries to take their own life but it doesn't happen for any reason then they are more susceptible to further attempts along with new or additional mental health disorders. A suicide attempt is never to be taken lightly, it should never be shrugged off, belittled or seen as a sign of weakness.

Those who attempt suicide might find themselves stuck in a more horrific place than they were before. A so-called 'failed attempt' can play over and over again in that person's mind until such time they believe suicide was the right answer all along.

Having failed to take one's own life can lead to life-changing mental health disorders and lifestyle changes. They should already be receiving mental health care for their suicide attempt. If they're not then it might be a good time to reach out to professionals for them.

Extreme Change in Eating Habits

This pertains to rapid weight loss or weight gain and generally cannot be explained by the person in question.

There's a difference between bulking up for the gym and gaining weight through over-eating. There's a difference between losing weight healthfully and consuming too little food that it becomes dangerous.

There can be healthy changes to eating habits but this section doesn't deal with the healthy side of it and you should be able to know the difference. Over one million people in the UK have eating disorders, also known as ED. It causes both physical and mental health problems and can also be a consequence of a mental health disorder.

It's important to realise that eating disorders affect so many people that it can come in so many different forms. ED doesn't just mean anorexia or bulimia, it can mean obesity and over-eating also. There's also a myth that eating disorders are limited only to females, they're not. It affects both sexes in the same way. We only hear about female ED because it is a more vocal community.

You can't just tell someone to eat less or eat more, it doesn't work like that. There are a thousand different reasons why someone might develop an eating disorder but mostly it is linked to some form of mental health issue. It can also be a sign of suicide as it is linked to one of the many methods than people choose to end their lives.

Act responsibly and with care around someone whose eating habits have changed dramatically. Seek to get to the core of the issue and always let them know that you are there for them, whatever happens.

We look deeper into eating disorders in the mental health disorders section.

Planning Signs

Suicide is never normally a spur of the moment decision, it has usually been thought about and planned with some effort beforehand. This is why it is important to notice the signs in order to save lives.

How does someone plan for suicide?

It's not like they have a checklist of items to tick off, it's mostly how they act or what they say that are the most telling signs. Most people **DO** plan suicide and they show very particular signs that they are at least thinking about it.

Here are some signs that might show someone is planning to take their own life.

Giving Away Possessions

This is as obvious as it is difficult to see. When someone gives away a lot of their own belongings or possessions then you have to question why they are doing it.

Are they giving up material items to make more space or to rearrange their living accommodation? That's okay!

Everyone needs a refresh from time to time, although it might be an idea to check to see if they're doing the right thing and if there is anything you can help with.

When we talk about giving away possessions as a warning sign of suicide, it's generally when people have no real reason to give up those possessions. If you have a friend who's been collecting Blu-ray for a decade and suddenly decides to give them away for free then it should sound off alarm bells.

If there's not a real and tangible reason then an assumption could be made that the person is getting rid of their possessions as part of a larger plan to take their own life. It doesn't matter what they give away or how inconsequential it may seem, there could be something bigger at work.

Any of the following possessions someone gives up could be a sign of active suicidal ideation.

- Private collections.
- Photo albums.
- Personal computer equipment.
- Kitchen items (microwave/toaster/kettle/grill)
- Jewellery.
- Expensive items they could normally sell on.
- An item they have owned since childhood.

- Gifts from family members and friends.
- Family keepsakes.
- Items that have sentimental value.

It's important to find out the real reason why they are giving up their possessions. If they are really planning suicide then they will be well-versed in deflecting attention away from the real reasons and try to palm you off with a soft excuse. Don't let them, keep digging and you will find the truth behind their actions.

This book shows you how to start up conversations and what questions to ask in the intervention section.

Putting Affairs in Order

Most people that have planned suicide will have gone through their own accounts, lifestyle, and personal affairs to get them in order beforehand. This means that they may have transferred any remaining bank funds to a family member's account or a charity.

It could also mean they pay off any debts owed and wrap up any business that needs wrapping up. It's mostly something that can only be carried out by themselves such as their personal accounts.

Putting affairs in order could look like any of the following:

- Paying off old debts to friends.
- Paying off personal or business debt.
- Transferring bank accounts to family or a charity.
- Wrapping up a business.
- Making amends with others unexpectedly.
- Writing or changing a will.
- Closing all personal accounts.
- Stopping all direct debits coming out of an account.
- Closing entertainment accounts such as Netflix or Amazon.
- Paying for their own funeral.
- Giving away possessions (previous section).

It's difficult to see what someone is doing with their own accounts but if you spot something similar to the above then it might be time to step in. If you are generally concerned then it is time to open up a conversation. We show you how in the intervention section.

Writing Goodbye Letters

Not to be confused with a suicide note which is usually one letter addressed to everyone or a particular named person.

A goodbye letter could look like any of the following:

- A thank you for helping or being there for them.
- Describing how it is too late to save them now.
- Arranging funeral costs.
- Discussing a will in the event of their death.
- That no one will miss them.
- Blaming others for what is about to happen.
- Talking about their own endgame.

It could be in the form of an:

- Email.
- Letter (snail-mail).
- Text.
- Social media message.
- A note pushed through your door.
- A note left in your pocket.

If a letter or message comes your way and it looks like a goodbye letter then you must take immediate action. Find out where they are and get to them. If you struggle to do it yourself then call the emergency services who will be at their door in a flash.

Don't leave it to chance in the hope that it was a one-off and will be better by morning. If someone has sent a goodbye letter then they could be close to taking their own life or be susceptible to a mental health disorder.

Other warning signs that have been linked to suicidal ideation include sleeping too much or too little and talking about being a burden to others.

It's important to not put other people down for their feelings or their expression of emotion. It's vital that we respect others, lift them up and praise them for everything they do right and guide them positively through a mistake they might make.

A mistake or a moment of bad behaviour does not define a person.

As soon as we can understand that then we can go some way to appreciating others more and allowing for certain behaviours that might be out of the ordinary.

Next up we look at the Risk Factors of suicide which are quite different from the warning signs.

Risk Factors

Risk factors are based around society, culture, ways of living, external and environmental influences. Warning signs are what someone might display when they are considering suicide as an option, whereas risk factors are usually out of their own control.

The major categories of risk factors include:

- Isolation & Social Inequality.
- Violence or abuse.
- Self-Harm.

Each section has its own sub-categories that go into detail and lists what the risk factors may look like in real life.

Isolation/Social Inequality

Isolation, self-inflicted or otherwise is one of the biggest reasons why people might move towards suicidal ideation. If a person cuts themselves off from the world then the only voice they listen to is the one in their head.

Once thought processes turn to the negative, as they undoubtedly will, then a greyness drops over the world and leaves them crying out for help in silence.

Silent screams are never heard.

There are routes to isolation that are as obvious as they are complicated and we take a look at a few of them below. If you know someone who you can allocate one or more of these risk factors to then it's time to open up the conversation.

Examples of what isolation might look like:

- Cutting all ties with family and friends.
- General lack of interest in anything.
- Loss of a spouse.
- Withdrawal from social life.
- Disinterest in work or activities.

- Hoarding at home.
- Developing poor eating habits.
- Disconnecting lines of communication.
- Becoming socially adverse.
- Fearful of the outside world and other people.
- Loss of self-esteem and confidence.
- Lack of important relationships.
- Losing means of transportation.
- Ageing.
- Victim of domestic violence.
- Skipping regular classes or activities.

A person isolating themselves are sometimes referred to as asocial. Asociality is when someone displays a lack of motivation to engage in social interaction or develops an interest in solitary activities.

Living On Benefits

There is a myth that most people on benefits are lazy and don't want to work. If you believe that then the media narrative has influenced you because it's not true, at least not always.

Sure, there are some people on benefits who abuse the system. They may have been born into the benefit system with a non-working or disabled family or they may have discovered that being on benefits brings its own – benefits.

Do we blame them? I'm sure most of us do to some degree. Our prejudices and knowledge are spoon-fed to us by those who would think themselves higher than another person. Yet, the truth of being on benefits is generally extremely far from the ten kids and aggressive drunks we've been led to believe.

The benefits system – if it works properly – is there to support those who cannot work for a multitude of reasons. Some of these reasons could include:

- Being made redundant.
- Physical accident.
- Mental health issues.
- Life-changing injury.
- Forced retirement.
- Retired military personnel.
- Escaping an abusive relationship.
- Being made homeless.
- Financial ruin.

Do we blame **them** for being on benefits? We shouldn't because they have every right to access the benefits system.

The difficulty comes when those people realise that they don't have what they had before.

If someone had been earning £30,000 a year in an office job and then through one of the reasons above they end up on benefits, it can be a lot to deal with. Some circumstances might result in that person losing their home, their car and their relationship. It could leave them in debt, struggling to survive and forced to look to food banks for help.

It leaves their mental health fractured and open to negative influence and damaging suggestion. It is a time when suicidal ideation might creep in and take hold when they least expect it. It's also a time when as a friend or family member you could be helping them get through it.

Living on benefits can be difficult, testing and crushing all at the same time. It can rip the self-esteem right out from inside of you and show it to the world for all to see.

It's only right that we look out for those who don't have as much as maybe we do. Living on benefits can sometimes go hand in hand with the next section.

"We live in this world together and without each other we are nothing at all."

Mentacracy: Living Under The Rule Of Mental Illness

Living In Poverty

Poverty is not necessarily linked with benefits, although a connection can sometimes be made. Even if you're working in the UK, earning £30,000 a year, you still might find yourself below the bread-line and struggling to feed your family or yourself.

- Firstly, income tax demolishes your salary, leaving you with an approximate £24,000.
- Your rent is £1,000 a month, leaving you at £12,000.
- Amenities and council tax bills come to £250 a month so that puts you down to £9,000. That sounds great but hold on a minute...
- You forgot about the £500 a month you need to fork out on food, car costs, travel to work, clothing and other shopping essentials. This leaves you £3,000 a year or £250 per month.
- £30,000 a year to £250 a month in a matter of seconds.
- You might want to get birthday gifts, a takeaway

> once a month, a drink in the pub with friends, or try and put some away, then you're left with nothing.

We need to get out of the mindset that someone earning more than us is going to be better off, it's not always true. If the person with the above example then suddenly needs to access the benefits system then everything becomes even more difficult.

Poverty can affect anyone from any walk of life, it's important to realise that just because someone earns more than another doesn't necessarily mean that they are wealthy or not struggling. Which again is why we need to reach out.

It is of course an exaggerated example but it's not too far from the truth of what happens day in day out. If you're on benefits then you too might end up with a couple of hundred quid after everything is paid and it's even tighter because you've got to pay for food out of it.

For a lot of people struggling financially or on benefits they find themselves on sprawling council estates that can be lively at any time of the day or night. Just living on an estate can be enough to push someone over the edge and consider suicide, especially if they are more open to negative influences.

People on lower income are **more likely** to act on suicidal tendencies.

Housing estates and projects are no longer the bastion of post-war era gangs and violence. There are still some estates where things do go wrong and it becomes difficult to live in but it has got better. Regardless, living on a rough estate and constantly hearing violence and feeling unease where you live can bring with it negative mental health issues.

One method of talking to someone who lives on an estate is to take the estate out of the equation.

Remove them from where they feel most uncomfortable and provide them with a safe space.

A safe place could look like any of the following:

- A bench in the park.
- Walk along a shoreline.
- An out-of-town family restaurant.
- A shopping centre.
- Countryside or forest walk.

Once they feel a bit safer or freer then allow them to open up and be there for them. Always assure the person that they are not alone and you are there to talk or listen at any time on any day.

A bit further into this book we look at examples of conversations you can have and questions you can ask.

Exposure To Suicide

One of the most over-looked areas of suicidal ideation is when an individual is exposed to the suicidal behaviour of others.

Psychologically, the more we are around people who are trying to take their own life or are exposed to news around suicide then the more likely we are to absorb those negative influences and act on them.

It's one of the reasons why counsellors and therapists have to take regular check-ups for their own mental health. Exposure to suicide is as dangerous to your own mental health as suicidal ideation itself.

There are various ways of being exposed to suicide and you might recognise at least one of the types of exposure below.

You could be exposed to suicide through:

- Anyone you knew who had taken their own life.
- Someone who has attempted suicide.
- A celebrity suicide.
- News about suicide and self-harm.
- Social media hashtags.
- Television programmes.

- Films that feature suicide.
- Certain music where lyrics talk about suicide.

As you can see, it's not just direct exposure to suicide, it can be indirect as well. We absorb all the information around us, sometimes without knowing. It can overwhelm and grind a person down so much that they start thinking about suicide in a negative way. This negativity feeds their mind and soon enough they might be looking at suicide in such a way that they need help themselves.

Exposure to suicide in itself can cause suicidal ideation. It's important we notice how it affects children who hear about it and how it affects the people around us. We should step in when we see that a person is affected by what they have directly or indirectly experienced.

Some think that media and policy makers should be held more accountable for poor reporting and poor discussion about mental health and suicide. Although it's easy to blame others, we all need to take responsibility for how we talk about suicide and mental health. We also need to know when to step in and turn the negative to the positive.

Isolation risk factors also include people who have been recently released from prison, feeling trapped in a certain way of life or struggling to feed themselves.

Violence Or Abuse

Being on the receiving end of violence or abuse is one of the leading risk factors of suicide. We look at some of the different types of abuse below.

Emotional or Psychological Abuse

Emotional abuse is one of the hidden and less-spoken about causes of mental illness and can be as devastating as physical abuse. Not only does it rip the self-esteem out of the person on the receiving end, but it can also lead to multiple mental health disorders, loneliness, and a withdrawal from the world.

The *ONS (Office for National Statistics)* still don't have a fully-fledged report on emotional abuse cases and consequences. Their domestic abuse reports are detailed and up-to-date as of March 2019. Yet, there are only a few lines that separate emotional abuse from more commonly known and understood types of domestic abuse.

In October 2018, the British Government's guidance on domestic abuse put emotional abuse at the top of the list for the first time. It was a glimmer of light that emotional abuse might be better understood in years to come.

Emotional abuse can come from anyone including parents, spouses, family members, friends, colleagues or random people in the street. There's a difference between jesting with friends and deliberately being psychologically abusive towards another person.

Here are some things that people say when they are knowingly or unknowingly using emotional abuse as a tool for control or belittlement.

- "You should be making more money."
- "The wedding ring you got me was cheap and pointless."
- "You're pathetic, why can't you do anything right?
- "Why can't you be like other men?"
- "If I split up with you then no one else will want you."
- "You're fat and ugly."
- "You're too unfit and you look unfit."
- "I'm buying your clothes from now on, you have bad fashion taste."
- "You've always made wrong decisions and you always will."
- "What's the point of you existing?"

Mostly, if someone who is meant to love you resorts to name-calling then it is a clear sign of emotional abuse.

Emotional abuse can also be expressed through actions such as:

- Arguments that are one-sided.
- Silent treatment.
- Shouting down another person.
- Being overly patronising.
- Embarrassing you in public.
- Belittling your successes.
- Threats of any form.
- Financial control.
- Treating you like a child.
- Jealousy.
- Dehumanisation.
- Indifference to your own feelings.

The list can be endless and can come in many forms that are individually tailored to the person on the receiving end. Some people who emotionally abuse others are not always aware they are doing it but they will appear as controlling people or those who are dismissive of another's needs.

Emotional abuse is silent, soul-destroying and deadly. There will be a noticeable change in a person receiving emotional abuse. It's also quite easy to see but most people dismiss it as a rift between partners or siblings and not for what it really is.

"We're not snowflakes or weak men, we simply have the esteem ripped out from us and crushed in our partner's hands."

Physical Abuse

Physical violence is a factor in family and home environments more than it is on the outside. Both can have a major impact that may lead to suicidal ideation. Violence towards a pet or animal can also be a trigger, as can witnessing a fatal or horrific accident.

An extraordinary incident can put ordinary people at risk.

Physical abuse is sometimes separated from sexual abuse even though sexual abuse is a form of physical abuse. In this instance we are talking about violence towards another person that is not primarily sexual in nature.

Children who are physically abused are at risk of developing social problems at a later stage in their life. They may also channel their own aggression towards others as a way of dealing with their own inability to fight back. The risk of suicide is extremely high among those who have experienced physical or sexual abuse.

When a child is abused in any way, they can't physically fight back and some might lean towards attacking small animals as an outlet.

This is because some animals such as cats can easily be overcome by the child. As they grow up and get physically bigger, they start becoming aggressive towards others in their own age group and so on and so forth.

Physical violence in childhood or at any age can lead to a person developing PTSD. Over 30% of children who experience abuse go on to become abusive as adults. If you notice a child has marks or has likely been abused then it is a human responsibility to step in, regardless of what you think the consequences might be.

Nothing positive has ever come from doing absolutely nothing when we see someone in need.

Types of physical abuse could look like any one of the following:

- Scratching or biting.
- Pushing.
- Slapping or hitting.
- Kicking
- Choking or strangulation.
- Throwing objects.
- Using weapons against you.

Other factors involved in physical violence are less talked about. They include intimidation from family members or friends. Intimidation is not purely physical, as a person can be psychologically threatening but they can also use their physical presence to intimidate you.

It also includes victims of violent crime. Whether it is a mugging or on the receiving end of alcohol-induced violence, it's all linked to physical abuse. Every person on the receiving end is likely to develop at least mild mental health issues, if not full-on suicidal ideation.

If your friend has been beaten up or attacked then don't leave them alone, they will be going through all kinds of different emotions and will need someone there for them.

On the other side of that, if a person has witnessed violence or threatening behaviour then they too might be at risk. We think we have been desensitised through violent films and aggressive music lyrics but we haven't. Our minds are quite aware that films or music are not always real life. It knows how to differentiate between the two.

This is why when we are witness to violence, it takes a higher emotional toll on us. The latest problem is that real violence has become rife on internet video channels and social media despite processes in place to stop them being made public.

The truth is that if you watch a violent video or see something disturbing then you're at higher risk of suicidal ideation and mental health issues. If these types of videos are popping up in your feed or on your channel then block the person who originally posted it.

There is no biological **NEED** to see an extreme act of violence or aftermath of a terrorist attack. You might wish to be aware of the facts and understand what happened but you don't really need to see it. There is no real human need to view violent acts beyond our own curiosity.

Sexual Abuse

The difference between emotional, physical, and sexual abuse is that during sexual abuse it is your entire body and soul that is being used and manipulated. Now before you skip this section because sexual abuse might be a bit grim, have a think about what sexual abuse really is because it's different than you might realise.

Sexual abuse is sickening but it also includes things that you might see in a pub or on the street and not have two thoughts about either way. There is no real scale of sexual abuse, save to say that rape or forced sexual relations are at the top of the pyramid.

Generally, as most of this normally is, it's male towards female. Biologically speaking it's because men have the means with which to penetrate a woman, and some might use this to a selfish advantage.

Men also suffer sexual abuse and it's one of those stigmas that is still so difficult to break.

Firstly, let's look at some things that are considered mild sexual abuse. Have a look at the following list and you might see some scenarios that look familiar or have happened to you. If some of the following seem tame to you then it's time to really start thinking about your actions.

- Slap on the bum.
- Nipple twists.
- Crotch grabbing.
- Someone rubbing up against you.
- Being forced to watch sexual intercourse.
- Unwarranted kissing.
- Hands constantly touching you.
- Someone touching your face.
- Being hugged too tightly.
- Someone putting their hand up your shirt.
- Stroking your hair against your will.

Now you've read that then consider this: What if everything in the list above was happening to a man by another man? Does it make you feel any different? If you're in pub and your mate slaps your bum as a friendly gesture you might think of it as being just what friends do.

Now what if the guy having his bum slapped is gay? Or maybe you don't know that your friend is gay and you've just sexually groped him. At the end of the day, it doesn't matter whose bum you slap, it can be considered sexual abuse. Your friend might take offence that you just touched them in a sexual manner regardless of whether you think it to be socially and culturally acceptable.

The above won't necessarily make someone take their own life but it might play over in their minds and potentially lead to mental health issues down the line. Unless you are in a physical relationship with someone then you really have no right to touch, grope, or squeeze them in a manner that could be seen as being overtly sexual.

On the other end of the spectrum of sexual abuse is rape and forced sexual contact. Children who are sexually abused are more likely to experience mental health problems and are a potential suicide risk at a young age and later in life. Some children bottle up their pain and keep it within them for years, pretending to fit in with society when all they wish for is a way out.

If someone is brave enough to tell you of sexual abuse they experienced as a child then be there for them. Listen to as much or as little as they want to discuss. The very act of talking about their abuse can be some form of therapy to them.

There are specialised therapy programmes and networks for children who have been abused and they should be contacted as a first port of call. If you are aware of a child being abused and nothing has already been done then call the police immediately. You might even save that child's life.

If a teenager or adult is raped then they are at a high risk of suicidal ideation. Rape is one of the most heinous acts another human being can do to another. Rape can happen from men to men, women to women, men to women, women to men and everything in-between.

Gay men are at a higher risk of being raped for many reasons. They might be privately gay and have not come out yet or believe that it was their own fault in many ways. In fact, many gay rapes happen in relationships and are hardly ever made public. It's difficult for anyone to report rape but for gay men it can be even more difficult because of societal taboos that still exist.

If you have a friend who has even made the tiniest insinuation that they have been sexually attacked then you have a right to step in and intervene. All rape victims are at an extremely high risk of self-harming and developing mental health issues. Again, there are specialised groups that help rape survivors and these are listed in the end matter of this book.

Self-Harm

Previous suicide attempts or people who self-harm are at extremely high risk of suicide. 16% of suicide survivors try again within a year with 2% of repeat attempts being fatal. Self-harm is only second to previous suicide attempts when looking at suicide statistics.

From April 2018 to April 2019, there were **114,091** cases of self-harm listed as a cause for admittance to an NHS hospital in the UK alone. The number includes those that may have been admitted or seen by a consultant more than once.

Let that sink in for a moment.

The figure of 114,091 is the amount of times registered **ONLY** in NHS hospitals. According to NHS digital, it does not include mental health care carried out in a non-hospital environment. It also doesn't include a large number of people who do not seek help for self-harm. That number is unknown.

As the 2019 to 2021 figures have not been completed, we can only go by snippets of the data revealed to the public. The snippets show that admittance to hospital for self-harm has doubled in certain age groups.

The age group with the highest number of self-harm admissions in hospitals was 15 to 24-years-old with **36,512** cases. In the 45 to 49-year-old range, which is where the most amount of suicides occur, the number was **8,618**.

There are different types of self-harm including direct and indirect. The next section goes into the reasons and risk factors to look out for.

Reasons For Self-Harm

Self-harm can be a cause or consequence of mental illness. If someone is self-harming then it doesn't mean they are about to end their own life. Self-harm can be an addiction like gambling, drink, or drugs and requires the same level of help to stop self-harming.

Some people might self-harm as practice for suicide while others do it because they become addicted to it or see it as a coping mechanism for various issues. There are many reasons why people self-harm and they are as individual as they are plentiful.

Although the reasons listed here don't always lead to self-harm they can be contributing factors. They can also be reasons that lead to other mental health issues and active suicidal ideation. If you know anyone that falls under one of the following risk factors then it's time to check in on them.

Traumatic Experiences

These could extend from childhood or occur in adult life. No-one is immune from trauma of any kind and so those who have suffered trauma recently should be checked in on more often than not.

- Loss of a loved one or pet.
- Childhood abuse.
- Domestic abuse of any kind.
- Life-changing accident.
- Sexual/physical abuse.
- Violence or threat to a person.
- Natural disaster.
- Experiencing war as a soldier or refugee.
- Onset of sudden illness.
- Witness to violence or accident.
- Exposure to violence or threat.

Bullying

There are two ways in which someone can bully another; online and in real life. Both are equally as traumatic or threatening and should be treated seriously. A lot of these risk factors are interchangeable with overall suicide risk factors but can lead to self-harm which can then lead to active suicidal ideation.

Some examples of bullying might include:

- Social media bullying and trolling.
- Social media threatening/belittling behaviour.
- Being bullied in school or college.
- Office and workplace bullying.
- Domestic abuse.
- Emotional or psychological abuse.
- Physical or sexual abuse.
- Physical intimidation and threats.
- Psychological intimidation and threats.
- Belittling behaviour or name-calling.

Sometimes it might feel as though the person being bullied cannot escape from their lives and might use self-harm or other methods to distract themselves.

Pressures

Some pressure can be healthy but negative pressure can come in all forms and types. Sometimes it can take over a person's life and become overwhelming if not dealt with.

Examples of negative pressure:

- Office and workplace pressure.
- Pressure in exams and in school.
- The pressure to have sex before you're ready.
- Spousal or relationship pressure.
- Pressure to be successful.
- Pressure to show others everything is good.
- Social media pressure.
- Pressure of expectation.
- Peer pressure; drink, drugs, or negative actions.
- Stress in all forms.

Risk factors of self-harm also include people who are put under undue stress which is sometimes linked to pressure. It also includes depression which we take a look at under the mental health disorders section.

Now let's look at the two types of self-harm and what they actually mean.

"Strong people don't put others down, they lift them up."

Michael P. Watson, former professional boxer

Direct Self-Harm

Direct self-harm means to take immediate action to physically hurt oneself. This is sometimes referred to as Non-suicidal self-injury (NSSI) and involves deliberate acts that damage the body but are not for the purpose of suicide.

Types of NSSI or direct self-harm could involve:

- Cutting.
- Burning.
- Scratching.
- Bruising.

Direct self-harm is what people think of the most when they hear the words; self-harm. It's difficult to get an image out of your head of someone taking a blade to themselves. It's an image that the media has shoved down our throats for decades.

There is also a myth that self-harm is an attempt at suicide but it's not always the case. Self-harm can be a warning sign of active suicidal ideation and it is one of the major risk factors. However, most self-harm is NSSI which as we found out above means it is non-suicidal self-injury.

There is no difference between self-harm and self-injury, both terms are interchangeable. You might read self-injury being used more commonly in North America and self-harm in Europe but either way they mean the same thing.

Direct self-harm can be dangerous and damaging to a person's health. The very act of direct self-harm means to deliberately hurt oneself. With some of the methods given above, the harm may be life-changing. The scars of direct self-harm can remain with someone for life.

For some, the scars become a reminder of how much strength it took to overcome self-harm. Some survivors of self-harm celebrate each year they have been free of it, in the same way that a former alcoholic would celebrate another year of sobriety.

There are those for whom the meaning of their scars is deeper and they find it difficult to overcome the feeling they had at the time they self-harmed. The scars are a daily reminder of every negative emotion and thought they ever had.

If someone is directly self-harming then they need immediate intervention and help. It's not good enough to stand by and watch someone cut themselves or provide them the means with which to do so. Self-harm is a pathway to mental illness or a result of mental illness. An exceedingly high percentage of people who self-harm don't just do it once, they hurt themselves on multiple occasions.

Indirect Self-Harm

Indirect self-harming is when people take part in activities that don't immediately hurt them. When we think of self-harm, usually we think of direct self-harm but indirect self-harm is rife and it's important to notice it.

Indirect self-harm is also based around non-suicidal behaviour but it doesn't directly damage the body with immediate effect.

Types of indirect self-harm:

- Involvement in abusive relationships.
- Constant drug abuse.
- Alcohol abuse.
- Overly risky or reckless behaviour.
- Eating disorders.
- Involving oneself in violence.

A study carried out in 2006 (*St Germain SA, Hooley JM)* showed that indirect self-harm did not always lead to mental health disorders but that addiction behaviours led to negative thought processes.

Direct self-harmers were more likely to see a significant increase in aggression, negative temperament, depressive symptoms and borderline personality disorder. They are also the type to be more self-critical and have a history of self-harming.

Both types of self-harm are seen as separate issues within the medical field but both still carry a huge weight in relation to how we understand mental health.

We listed involvement in an abusive relationship as one of the types of indirect self-harm. You might be wondering why? Some people, whether they were abused as a child or not, seek out controlling partners as a way to submit to another. The notion of submission isn't purely sexual but one in which a person hands over control of their life to another.

We sometimes wonder why people do not leave an abusive relationship and it's not always to do with fear. They might actively seek out partners who are abusive as a way to have others punish them where they cannot punish themselves.

Nothing positive comes out of an abusive relationship. If you know someone, male or female, who is in a dangerous relationship whether held captive by fear or control then you need to look at all options to get them out. We look at ways of starting conversations in the intervention section.

Mental Health Disorders

At its core, this book is about mental health. Many people who suffer from mental illness before being diagnosed had no idea they were suffering from a mental illness.

It's the most important thing to learn from this book. Some people do not know they are mentally ill and this is down to a lack of knowledge and understanding.

In hindsight, people know more about mental health **after** their diagnosis than before. That's what we need to change as a society to really make a difference.

What if we could turn the tables? What if we could teach people to be aware of mental health before they ever come across it? The consequence of this knowledge is that more people will be prepared to deal with negative emotions and thoughts long before a mental disorder ever takes hold.

What does that have to do with this book? Everything you learn in here; the warning signs, risk factors, myth busters, mental health, self-help and the rest, combine to make a powerful psychological arsenal to help yourself and others.

This book is arming you with the knowledge to go out and save lives. It's down to **you** as an individual to do this.

"My life amounts to no more than one drop in a limitless ocean. Yet what is any ocean, but a multitude of drops?"

Cloud Atlas by David Mitchell.

Types of mental disorders include:

- Depression.
- Acute/Psychotic Depression.
- Schizophrenia.
- Dementia.
- Anxiety Disorders.
- Eating Disorders (ED)/Body Dysmorphia (BD).
- Post-Traumatic Stress Disorder (PTSD).
- Borderline Personality Disorder (BPD).
- Obsessive Compulsive Disorder (OCD).

There are many more but most are associated with the above list. We'll take a look at some of those in the following sections.

Mood Disorder

Depression is the most common but least understood of the mental disorders. There's a big difference between feeling down and suffering from depression.

When you feel down, you might feel pissed off with the world, upset with yourself or saddened by another person's actions. It's not uncommon to feel sad or upset, it is a human emotion and one that can be used in a positive way.

Being sad doesn't make you depressed, it makes you human.

We can feel down for a variety of reasons and it's okay to feel that way, we all feel a little sad sometimes. Does crying at a movie make you someone who is suffering from depression? No, it makes you human, just like anyone else.

Some major depressive episodes lead to extreme delusions, hallucinations, dissociation with reality and internal voices and that's just the start of it. Bear in mind that there are many types of depression and many ways it can take hold.

Types Of Depression

Major depression

Major depression, also known as major depressive disorder, is one of the more common examples of depression. Millions of people a year suffer from major depression or experience a major depressive episode.

People with major depression show symptoms on a daily basis. They may appear to be living a normal life but internally they might be struggling day in and day out. As with all depression, it's one of the hardest to spot from afar which is why I've expanded the depression sections to give you a better understanding of what it really is and what to look out for.

Symptoms of major depressions include:

- Grief, in all its forms.
- Loss of hope.
- Constantly worrying.
- Sleeping problems, either too little or too much.
- Lack of energy.
- Lack of motivation.

- Eating problems, under or over-eating.
- Unexplained aches or pains anywhere on the body.
- Lack of concentration.
- Loss of memory.

These symptoms can last weeks or even months. Some people might have a single episode of major depression, while others experience it throughout their life. Regardless of how long its symptoms last, major depression can cause problems in relationships and daily activities.

Bipolar disorder

Bipolar disorder is one of the more common diagnoses when it comes to depression. It used to be called manic depression but thankfully we have come through the era when mental health was ridiculed and frowned upon.

Bipolar is when someone can be up or down at any particular time. The moods range from being extremely energetic and happy to being depressed and slow-moving. Those who suffer from bipolar will exhibit all the signs of major depression when they are at their lowest.

It is a disorder that is misunderstood both in the public eye and from the media. Someone suffering from it will appear to be completely normal and happy at one moment and then completely down and depressed the next. It's the extent of the mood swings that determine how extreme the disorder is affecting the individual.

Medication is the primary method of controlling the low mood swings but as you'll see in forthcoming chapters, there are other ways to take back control of a mental health disorder.

Seasonal Affective Disorder (SAD)

This is a disorder which usually affects people in the Winter months and arises due to a decrease in sunlight throughout the day. It's sometimes connected to the lack of Vitamin D our bodies have, which mostly comes from exposure to sunlight.

It's why you hear people talking about taking Vitamin D supplements in the Winter as a way to maintain their mood and feel happier. It would be wrong to say that Vitamin D improves depression because it doesn't but studies have shown it does have some minor benefits to assist with mood.

Seasonal Affective Disorder mostly goes away when the days become longer and the sunlight comes back from the Spring to the Summer. It's another reason why some people feel down on a cloudy or rainy day.

Psychotic Depression

This is a nasty disorder that pulls in elements from other mental health disorders. It is mostly a combination of a major depressive episode with elements of psychosis.

Psychotic depression is classified as a major depressive disorder with the addition of hallucinations, delusions and paranoia. It can though extend far beyond general delusions, such as believing in a conspiracy, and can eat away at a person's reality until they feel as though there is nothing left.

Hallucinations are generally on the extreme end of psychosis, with delusions being the most common. There is usually a belief that someone or something is out to get them. Having delusions combined with major depression can be controlled but it might take a much larger intervention in order to really make a difference.

Peripartum/Postpartum Depression

This can affect females in the months leading to and following on from giving birth. Both peripartum and postpartum are interchangeable words that are used to describe this particular type of depression.

Other types of depression can be episodic in nature and are the result of a situation or moment, sometimes referred to as 'situational depression'. It can stem from grief, sadness, anxiety, a difficult situation or many other circumstances. It is generally limited to a period of time.

Psychotic Disorder

It's important to note that psychotic depression is interchangeable both as a major depressive and a psychotic disorder. If psychotic depression is an ugly disorder then schizophrenia can be even worse.

People with psychotic disorders specifically show signs of delusions and hallucinations.

Schizoaffective Disorder

Usually known as schizophrenia. There's a common misconception that schizophrenia means to have multiple personalities but it doesn't. A person can never deliberately create multiple personalities, it's biologically impossible.

Schizophrenia is a psychotic disorder that combines hallucinations, delusions, major depression and a disconnection from reality. Someone who is schizophrenic will display signs of slowness both mentally and physically. They may appear to be completely disconnected from reality and you might struggle to have a conversation with them. But it doesn't mean you shouldn't.

People with schizophrenia need support, without it their lives would be much harder. Support comes in the form of friends, family, mental health workers and psychiatrists.

People with schizophrenia are no more dangerous than any other person.

Anxiety Disorders

Anxiety is one of the most common forms of mental disorder but it doesn't have to be all negative. Having some anxiety can be good for us, it can help us avoid danger. Just as in depression, there are normal levels of anxiety and there are abnormally high levels.

Feeling anxious

Everyone feels anxious every now and again, it's a feeling that might help us through a situation or make sure we're not falling into any danger. Normal anxiety feels like sitting on the edge of a bungee jump platform ready to dive off. It's called 'feeling anxious'.

Now imagine that feeling lasts for hours on end; that's high-level anxiety.

Suffering from anxiety

As you can see there is a big difference between being anxious and suffering from anxiety. It doesn't go away without help but they are relatively easy ways to treat it if we look at mental health disorders as a whole.

Mild medication, psychological self-help tools, distraction exercises, mindfulness and grounding techniques are some of the ways to control an anxiety attack.

Like most mental disorders, anxiety can grip anyone at any time for any reason, there is no single cause of anxiety, it is entirely down to the individual's situation. However, the symptoms of anxiety can look common in people who suffer from it.

Symptoms of anxiety include:

- lack of concentration.
- Sleeping problems.
- Feeling tired all the time.
- Inability to carry out normal tasks.
- Feeling nervous.
- Feeling weak.
- Restless and tense.
- Catastrophising.
- A belief that danger is nearby.
- Immense panic.
- Sweating uncontrollably.
- Hyperventilating (breathing heavily and rapidly).
- Increased and fast heart rate.

Catastrophising means to view or talk about an event or situation as worse than it actually is. Many of us catastrophise and it's a difficult frame of mind to get out of. It could be something as simple as cooking a meal and thinking about how bad it might be instead of how good it could be. Or it could lead to worrying about anything and everything **before** something happens.

Studies have shown that women are more likely to develop anxiety than men and it's never been made entirely clear why. Men suffer from anxiety too, so much so that we still find it difficult to talk about.

There is a misconception that anxiety makes men appear to be weaker than others. We tend to only hear about female anxiety but male anxiety is a real thing and is happening more often.

Anxiety affects people's day to day activities. It makes work and socialising difficult. Anxiety can also stop people leaving their home, in an effort to avoid stressful situations. It can affect a person's life so much that they might be more susceptible to other mental health disorders.

"If we can learn to understand one another then we can make a real difference in the world."

Personality Disorders

It's important to point out that people with personality disorders and/or schizophrenia are no more dangerous than your best friend or family member. There are many stigmas that still need to be smashed when we discuss personality disorders.

Personality disorders are among the most controversial of the mental health disorders simply because they are so poorly misunderstood that we believe them to be something else. Horror entertainment and stories of historical asylums tell us that personality disorders are defined by maniacal killers and evil monsters.

We don't live in a world of mythical monsters and Jekyll and Hyde characters, we live in the real world. Our world is a can of beer, Netflix and chill.

Mild personality disorders

Every person is unique and we all have personalities that are individual to us, no-one on the planet is exactly the same and that goes for identical twins; there's always a very minor difference. There are many personality types and how these personalities work.

We are defined by culture, society, peers, family, upbringing, what we eat and what we watch. We absorb the world around us. These differences are normal because they are what makes each and every one of us unique and diverse.

Personality disorders are harder to diagnose because everyone is so unique. We can't blame another person for behaving a certain way due to their personality type. We should not be discriminating against others because their personality type doesn't fit in with how we perceive the world.

Having a personality disorder means to have a pattern of extreme opinion or behaviour that makes it difficult to function within perceived normal parameters. It is difficult for that person to change their behaviour and they will find it near impossible to adapt to different situations. Work will be difficult as will having positive relationships with others.

Fundamentally, it is an influence of their personality that is extreme enough to alter multiple areas of their day to day life. Mostly, people develop personality disorders in the formative years.

Dissociative identity disorder (DID)

DID is a nasty mental disorder that can completely up-end someone's life. It also has the unfortunate stigma of having previously been called 'multiple personality disorder'. As you've seen in the schizophrenia section, no-one can deliberately create multiple personalities within their minds, it's impossible to do so.

DID is generally characterised by the maintenance of at least two distinct and relatively enduring personality types. It's difficult to diagnose because other personality disorders are displayed by changing behaviour and the inability to adapt.

It can be accompanied with memory loss, depression, self-harm and other self-injury methods such as substance abuse. DID is generally associated with extreme traumas, especially child abuse.

Borderline personality disorder (BPD)

In some countries, BPD is also known as 'Emotionally Unstable Personality Disorder' (EUPD). It is far more common than DID, which is usually exhibited after suffering an extreme trauma.

Borderline personality disorder is when someone suffers from long-term instability, mostly in their personal life. They may have a widely varying view of themselves and are prone to having strong emotional reactions to certain events or situations.

BPD is strongly associated with major depression as most sufferers feel the same hopelessness and dissociation that depression brings. BPD sufferers are more prone to active suicidal ideation and it's not really clear why except that it feeds into other mental health disorders in a negative way.

It can affect people whose family members may have suffered, leading to a belief that BPD may be genetic. Mostly, BPD begins in the teenage years and into early adulthood and is caused by any type of challenging situation.

Eating Disorders

Another misconception is that eating disorders only affect women and again it's not true. More females are indeed susceptible to eating disorders but males also suffer from anorexia, bulimia and binge-eating.

Some eating disorders can be hereditary and passed down from a family member who has suffered, but research is still being carried out in this field. Personality disorders can also cause eating disorders.

Seeking assumed perfection is another cause that is becoming more commonplace in our society. There is constantly talk and criticism aimed at magazines, news, and entertainment about showing female perfectionism which is mostly unattainable.

But what about men?

Look at any men's magazines (not those ones!) and you'll see cover after cover of athletic, ripped, muscly, perfect-looking men. No one really complains because it would be an assumed sign of weakness for a man to point it out. Seeking perfection is a human curse, not purely a specific gender one. An ideal body-type also changes with different cultures.

A study carried out in 2003 (*Keel PK, Klump KL*) showed that Western culture, which had been more exposed to the perfect body type, were more susceptible to eating disorders. Those cultures where exposure to 'perfection' was minimal were less likely to suffer from eating disorders.

Anorexia

There's a difference between trying to lose weight and dangerous weight loss caused by an eating disorder. Females suffer more from anorexia for a multitude of reasons include some of the causes given above. Men suffer too and it's a dangerous disorder that has the potential to become irreversible.

It's also known as **Anorexia Nervosa** and is the most well-known eating disorder. Those who don't understand Anorexia tend to be ignorant towards sufferers, which despite large awareness campaigns, still happens today.

Anorexia tends to start in the late teenage years and into adulthood. Some of the signs are as physical as they are mental. Most sufferers will be constantly checking their weight, avoiding most food types, dangerously cutting calories and also suffer from the belief that they are overweight when they are not.

Signs of Anorexia include:

- Being underweight.
- Not eating full meals.
- Limiting the number of times per day they eat.

- Constantly checking their weight.
- Striving towards a dangerous weight goal.
- Possible Body dysmorphic disorder (BDD)
- Unwillingness to be healthy.
- Weight denial.
- Low self-esteem.
- Lack of confidence or social skills.

Body dysmorphic disorder (BDD), also known as body dysmorphia, is a mental health disorder where people overly worry about their appearance or a certain part of their body. Mostly linked to personality disorders, it can sometimes be a cause or consequence of eating disorders.

Bulimia

Bulimia Nervosa, as it's also known, is another common eating disorder that is sorely misunderstood. The signs can be similar to that of Anorexia and usually begin in the teenage to adult years. Bulimia is more common in women but does affect men.

Signs of bulimia include:

- Consuming large amounts of food.
- Binge-eating.

- Lack of control over how much food is eaten.
- Eating food they would normally avoid.
- Forced vomiting to purge the consumed calories.
- Throwing up to relieve discomfort in the stomach.
- Taking laxatives.
- Fear of gaining weight.
- Low self-esteem.
- Excessive exercise.

Those with bulimia tend to stay a relatively healthy weight and don't usually become Anorexic. Bulimia can though lead to multiple health problems. The very act of forced vomiting in itself is dangerous not least to the stomach but for mental health as well.

It can also have negative effects on the lining of the throat, the glands and tooth enamel due to the acid being forced back up. It might also result in severe dehydration due to the vomiting of liquids and can have wide-ranging effects on hormonal levels.

Binge-eating

Binge-eating is different from bulimia because the sufferers tend not to forcibly vomit food back up. A binge-eating disorder can develop at any time in life from a teenager to people over 60-years-old. Some symptoms are similar to bulimia except the sufferers tend to be overweight.

They also exhibit a lack of control on food consumption and may eat large amounts in one sitting. Binge-eaters do not vomit or exercise to excess in order to remove their body of calories.

Pica

A rather less common eating disorder is known as Pica. It's a disorder that involves the consumption of items that are not considered food. People with Pica might eat items such as soil, soap, coal, hair, cardboard, paper, powders and man-made materials. It's a disorder that is commonly found in pregnant women, young children, or those already suffering from a mental disorder.

Trauma Related Disorders

Almost all trauma-related disorders are caused by a traumatic incident or overly stressful event. The signs of trauma-related disorders are generally emotional and behavioural.

Post-Traumatic Stress Disorder (PTSD)

It is the most commonly known of the trauma-related disorders. There is a misconception that PTSD only affects military or soldiers who have witnessed war. Yes, it can affect soldiers but PTSD is more commonly being seen in a wide-ranging segment of society and it is caused by many things.

PTSD usually lasts for more than one month and may not develop until at least six months after a traumatic experience.

Signs of PTSD include:

- Depression.
- Witness to a traumatic event.
- Anxiety.
- Fearful of everyday situations.
- Jumpiness.
- Sleep problems.
- Substance abuse.
- Headaches.
- Other physical aches, usually caused by stress.
- Nightmares.
- Distress.
- Withdrawal from society.
- Disinterest in daily activities.
- Disconnection from reality.

The type of traumas that lead to PTSD include any event or situation where a person experiences an overwhelming feeling of fear, helplessness, or horror. These could include serving in the military, sexual attack, abuse, terrorism, or even natural disasters.

PTSD is more common than you might think and can arise from any stressful situation or event. It can be a direct trauma or indirect trauma such as something happening to a loved one or having witnessed something horrific.

Almost 10% of people are affected by some level of PTSD in their lifetimes and is usually something that follows on from Acute Stress Disorder (ASD).

Acute Stress Disorder (ASD)

The difference between ASD & PTSD, is that ASD usually lasts for just a few days and up to a month. PTSD is long term and ASD is short-term.

The symptoms are fairly similar to PTSD with the exception of the length of time someone is experiencing symptoms for. ASD is caused by a direct or indirect traumatic experience and affects the individual's emotions and behaviour.

If symptoms of ASD last for longer than a month then they are diagnosed with PTSD which is an extension of ASD. We all experience stressful situations in our life and it's important to realise that some stress is good for us. It can help with pressure, challenges, overcoming fears and balance our emotions.

There is however a fine line between a small amount of stress and experiencing stress as a trigger for developing acute stress disorder.

Because we are all individuals, there are many types of stresses that some of us find easy to deal with that others will struggle with. Some people witness a traumatic event and it doesn't affect them but it doesn't mean they are stronger because they are not affected.

We all express emotions and behaviours differently from others, it's what makes us unique. We all experience varying levels of stress at different times in our lives and may see different consequences from it. ASD is to be taken as seriously as PTSD because just like PTSD it can be overwhelming and life-changing.

More than 90% of suicides and suicide attempts are found to have been associated with a mental health disorder. The most common denominator is depression but other mental disorders can also be a factor. There are many other illnesses and disorders that one might suffer from that lead off of the main categories listed here.

Mental illness can sometimes be a consequence of surviving a suicide attempt which is where noticing the signs can go some way to help preventing it. When a patient leaves intensive mental health care, they too might be more at risk due to the transition of acute care to a lesser level of care.

"To be yourself in a world that is constantly trying to make you something else is the greatest accomplishment."

Ralph Waldo Emerson, American philosopher and poet

More Risk Factors

We've looked at the main risk factors as to why someone might consider active suicidal ideation but there are many more that can influence a person's thoughts and emotions.

Some of them are cultural or societal and can affect people differently. The following list is made of up risk factors that might lead to one of the mental health disorders shown on previous pages.

Other risk factors include:

- Certain religious beliefs.
- Unemployment.
- History of abuse.
- Imprisonment/arrest.
- Unemployment.
- Family breakdown.
- Divorce.
- Relationship breakdown.
- Chronic pain.
- Some medical conditions.

- Family history of suicide.
- Owning guns/firearms.
- Exposure to celebrity suicide.
- Financial loss.
- Business pressures.
- Financial crisis/debt.
- Low self-esteem.
- Aggressive tendencies.
- Influence of suicide epidemics.

People react or view certain situations differently than others so it's important to consider not just the risk factors but the warning signs as well.

A knowledge of the warning signs and risk factors will put you in a better position to be able to save yourself or another.

"Don't fear mental illness, face it with confidence and calmness and you will prevail."

Intervention

Now that you're aware of the warning signs and risk factors, you are in a better place to understand when and if you should intervene in someone's life.

How, is a different matter altogether.

It's easy to say that because someone is displaying signs of depression that we will go and talk to them but it rarely happens. Humans are social animals who mostly protect themselves over others. It's difficult to really embed ourselves in another's life purely for their own benefit.

It's not good enough to ask how they are anymore, we need to spark up real conversations with real people in order to make a difference in society. In these sections, we'll look at social intervention, personal intervention, conversation starting points and real-world questions you can ask.

If suicide was easy to prevent then thousands of people each year in the UK would still be with us. Yet, there are preventive measures that can be taken and learned. The more we talk about them, the more lives we can save.

Social Intervention

Social intervention is something that those in authority could be helping to implement. Strategies range from education to task force groups.

Mental health education

At a fundamental level there needs to be mental health education in schools. In the same way that physical education (PE) is mandatory, so should mental health education (ME) also be mandatory.

Most people who succumb to a mental health crisis are unaware of what is happening to them and don't know what to do or where to turn. They might feel as though something is wrong with them but that it couldn't possibly be a mental health issue.

If people are made aware through education; the causes, consequences and self-help tools available to them then they would already be in a better position to help themselves.

Mental health education needs to become part of the national curriculum. If education at a primary level is introduced then at least the next generation would be better placed to understand and deal with mental health.

It's only right that we imbibe the next generation with our knowledge so that the current tsunami of mental health issues becomes more of a lapping wave on the shoreline of our future.

Social media restrictions

The internet changed our lives and social media changed it again.

In the past two years, social media platforms such as Twitter, Facebook, and Instagram have implemented measures of control when it comes to certain search terms.

Type in #selfharm or #suicide to Instagram for example and you'll be met with the following:

"Can we help? Posts with words or tags you're searching for often encourage behaviour that can cause harm and even lead to death."

After that they offer a link to get support. Twitter provides a call to action to contact the Samaritans. These are all steps in the right direction. Further restrictions could include social media limitations on age, usage, location filtering (such as not being able to use social media in schools) and more powerful content moderation.

In some instances, social media users have been linked with people who take their own lives. Bullying, trolling and attacking others online has led to devastating results.

Blame doesn't entirely rest with the social media networks, it rests with the users and the culture of false anonymity that has sprung up around social media. It's easy to tap buttons on laptops or phones but those same people probably wouldn't say the same things in person in the real world.

Social media can be good but it can also be bad. It's about finding the right balance to protect vulnerable people while at the same time giving others enjoyment on the platform of their choice.

Interventions by authorities

To improve the ways in which we intervene, there should be an introduction of a national system where people can report suicidal behaviour alongside improvements in current reporting methods.

There should be more investment in mental health services and awareness campaigns and more funding of counselling organisations. With increased access to community groups, there will be a higher percentage of people finding the help they need.

Other authority intervention possibilities include:

- Targeted surveillance of high-risk individuals.
- Reducing access to over-the-counter pharmaceuticals
- A proper database connection between authorities.

Targeted surveillance sounds pretty scary for people worried about privacy in the 21st Century but if it saved lives it might be seen as acceptable. Only time would tell if it was more acceptable or less acceptable than security services surveilling potential terrorist targets. It's a tricky scenario that could help or hinder saving lives.

As individuals, we should be raising awareness of mental health and actively reaching out to others. Governments of the world could also be doing a lot more and they should be doing a lot more. Other social intervention techniques include:

- Sponsored training for professionals.
- Reducing domestic violence.
- Reducing alcohol and drug abuse.
- Reducing access to the means of suicide.
- Reducing access to the methods of self-harm.
- Reducing the quantity of pills in boxes of painkillers.
- School-based curriculum education inclusion.
- Interventions of those at high risk.
- Surveillance systems targeted at high-risk groups.
- Implementation of social media restrictions.
- Improvements of how to report suicidal behaviour.
- Improving understanding of mental illness.

It's important to understand social intervention because it provides us with the tools and resources to use when we need to help others. It gives us a starting point where we can find the right help quickly and safely.

Personal Intervention

At a basic level, simply talking about mental health is as good a level of mental health awareness and intervention as any.

Too many people nowadays are still suffering alone and there's a good reason for it. People simply do not know where to turn for help and if they do then they struggle to reach out.

Most people who are suffering from a mental disorder or displaying warning signs of active suicidal ideation are simply unaware of what they are going through. It's as if the world has turned against them, delusions may come into play and they think that what is happening has happened to no other person.

This is where **YOU** as an individual can step in. Armed with the knowledge in this handbook, you can reach out and save a life.

You've read about the warning signs and the risk factors. You now have the knowledge to understand why someone might experience a mental health crisis or think of taking their own life.

The question then becomes; how?

How can you save someone's life?

Being knowledgeable of the warning signs and risk factors can already put you into a position of saving lives. You're now armed with the knowledge necessary to reach out, and now it's time to intervene.

The next sections show you:

- How to reach out.
- What to say.
- How to have a conversation.
- How to protect yourself.
- When to intervene.

"Tolerance leads to understanding.

Understanding leads to kindness."

Conversation Starters

What you say and how you say it can affect how a conversation plays out. Here you will find different types of conversation starting points so that you feel comfortable, knowing you're not going to offend someone or make them feel worse than they are already are.

In the next section we look at opening conversations with questions but you can start a conversation without asking questions. A question normally follows a conversation starter so it's good to know how to get one going.

Despite the rise of mental health advocates and online campaigners there is still stigma attached to actually talking about mental health. Throughout this section the aim is to get you talking about yourself or to others easily and with no worries about being rude or ignorant.

The next pages show some examples of conversation starters (CS) with someone who is feeling down or suffering from mental health issues.

- "I'm here for you, whatever you need, whenever you need it, I'm here."
- "You're not alone and I want you to know that."
- "Remember that you were not put on this world to suffer in silence."
- "We were given a voice so that we could converse with others.
- "I'd be more than happy to talk or listen for as long as you need."
- "A bad mistake or moment of bad behaviour does not define who you are as a person."
- "Try not to let the negative outweigh the positive."
- "Just talking to another person like me can go a long way to airing your problems and getting them off your chest."

- "No one should keep their problems to themselves.
- "We're all here for one another."
- "I've got time to talk."
- "I'm not going anywhere."
- "I hate to see you struggling alone."
- "Take as long as you need."
- "Remember when you were there for me?"
- "Let's solve this together."
- "You are the most perfect you there is."
- "I don't understand but I really want to, if you can talk to me then we can get through this together."
- "You do a lot for others but now is the time to take care of yourself."
- "Helping in any way I can is the most important thing right now."

Things NOT to say

There is a right way of sparking up a conversation and a wrong way to do it. Unfortunately, a lot of the wrong things to say are embedded into society as being the **RIGHT** things to say. This is where conversations can go wrong and fire up negative emotions on both sides.

Try **NOT** to say anything from the following list.

DON'T SAY:

"You shouldn't kill yourself because it will affect other people."

OR: *"Just think of all the people you'll leave behind."*

WHY?

It's tantamount to a **guilt trip**. Suicidal people require love, help and assistance, there's no need to make them feel guilty. Telling them about other people they will leave behind is not the right way to approach a conversation. The focus should be on them and not peripheral lives.

DON'T SAY:

"You'll get over it."

WHY?

It assumes that what they are going through is not important or is easy to overcome. The truth is, it's exactly the opposite. By belittling someone's struggles, we stop them talking deeper about their feelings.

DON'T SAY:

"It's only sadness."

OR: *"You're just sad, that's all."*

WHY?

Sadness is **NOT** depression. Everyone can feel sad or upset at something in their lives or a situation they experience but it doesn't make them depressed. Depression is a mental health disorder. Sadness is a human emotion all of us experience.

DON'T SAY:

"There's probably some quick fix to help you."

WHY?

There is no quick fix. Mental health is not normally cured, rather it is maintained. To say there is a quick fix is to be ignorant of the issues someone is facing.

DON'T SAY:

"Cheer up!"

OR: *"Put a smile back on your face."*

WHY?

You might not know what they are going through or have experienced. The very act of making oneself happy is not possible for a lot of people. If someone is suffering from depression, telling them to cheer up is to be ignorant of the issues they may be facing. It tells them that you don't really want to dig deeper and believe there is an easy way out.

DON'T SAY:

"It's all in your head."

WHY?

Mental health issues do affect the mind, that is true. Yet, telling someone it is all in their head means that you believe they can just snap out of it when they really can't. There are always deeper issues at the heart of mental health and it's never easy to simply snap out of it or brush it to one side.

DON'T SAY:

"You have a great life, you're always happy!"

WHY?

A lot of people mask their mental health issues and wear masks so they can function normally in the world. Although someone might appear to be happy doesn't necessarily mean that they are. To assume their world is perfect when they are clearly not feeling that way, makes them think that you will never understand what they are going through.

DON'T SAY:

"Everything is going to be okay."

WHY?

Chances are it probably won't be. It's okay to reassure but without understanding everything they are going through then it is more of uneducated assumption. It shows that you might be ignorant to their real issues.

DON'T SAY:

"You're only like this because it's the trend right now."

WHY?

Really not the right thing to say in anyway at all. Mental health issues are not spoken about because it's trendy or fashionable to do so, they are spoken about to raise awareness so that others may talk more freely. Mental illness is never trendy and is never a choice.

DON'T SAY:

"What you're talking about doesn't make any sense."

WHY?

You should avoid denying their feelings or emotions. They may be existing in a version of reality that you might not understand. It is best to avoid criticising or blaming that person for what they are going through.

DON'T SAY:

"Stop focusing on the bad stuff and get back in the world."

WHY?

This too is denying their feelings or emotions. You are assuming they can easily overcome the 'bad stuff' in their life by just swiping it to one side. That 'bad stuff' might be deep-rooted or might be the consequence of a mental disorder that is destroying their life both directly and indirectly.

The best thing to do is to show **respect** and **kindness** to the person you are talking to. Even if you do say one of the things above, you can always backtrack and apologise for not understanding what they are going through.

Direct Questions

Here you'll find a list of direct questions that you can ask without offending someone or worrying about how they might respond. Some might appear to be mundane or even similar to each other but they can all be leading points into a conversation about mental health.

Direct questions involve asking a person about themselves or their immediate surroundings. It enables them to talk about themselves and how they might be feeling at any given moment.

You can use any word in place of 'friend' as you would normally speak to a friend.

For example if we look at the first question:

(Q) Am I alright to chat for a few minutes?

You can add your style of talking after the fact, such as:

(Q) Am I alright to chat for a few minutes, MATE?

(Q) Am I alright to chat for a few minutes, BUDDY?

Two questions **NOT** to ask:

- (Q) How are you?
- (Q) How are you feeling?

They are quite simply **lazy** opening questions that are used too much and don't lead to a proper conversation. The most common replies from the above two questions will be one of the following:

- (A) Alright, thanks.
- (A) Not too bad.
- (A) So, so.
- (A) Could be better.
- (A) Meh!

You want someone to open up about what they are feeling or what they are going through. You don't want to ask one generic question, get a so-so answer and walk away.

Here is a list of direct questions that you can ask someone to open up a conversation about mental health and how they are feeling.

- (Q) Am I alright to chat for a few minutes?
- (Q) Would you like to talk about anything?
- (Q) Anything worrying you?
- (Q) How can I help?
- (Q) Do you have something you want to get off your chest?
- (Q) Could you tell me what you're feeling right now?
- (Q) Are you up to anything right now?
- (Q) What are you doing at the moment?
- (Q) Can I help you talk about things?
- (Q) What's on your mind?
- (Q) Are you having bad thoughts?
- (Q) What kind of thoughts are you having?
- (Q) What are you worried about the most?
- (Q) What do you think will happen?
- (Q) Could you be honest with me for a little bit?
- (Q) Can you talk to me about things?
- (Q) Would you talk to me about yourself?
- (Q) What are you thinking at the moment?
- (Q) Are you struggling?
- (Q) Is it okay if I start talking about mental health?
- (Q) When was the last time you spoke to someone

properly?

- (Q) Do you find it difficult to talk about your emotions?
- (Q) Would it be alright if I talk to you right now?
- (Q) How are you coping with things?
- (Q) Do you remember the last time you felt like this?
- (Q) Have you ever spoken to someone about what you're feeling?
- (Q) If I ask you how you're feeling will you be honest with me?
- (Q) Will you let me know if there is anything I can do to help?
- (Q) Any chance you could tell me what you're struggling with?
- (Q) How about having a one-to-one conversation so we can both open up?
- (Q) If I was suffering, would you leave me alone?
- (Q) If you saw someone else in pain, what would you do?
- (Q) Did you know that talking about your problems really does help?
- (Q) Looks like you have a lot to carry (mentally), can I offer some help?
- (Q) Would you be comfortable planning a time and place where we could have a life chat?

Indirect Questions

Here you'll find a list of indirect questions that you can ask without offending someone or worrying about how they might respond. As with direct questions, some might appear to be mundane or obvious but they can help open people up to conversational therapy.

Indirect questions are those that don't directly involve a person or their immediate surroundings. The idea behind indirect questioning is to open up a line of communication which can lead into direct questions.

If you can open up a line of conversation then you are in an easier place to talk about their feelings and emotions when you feel the time is right. It helps them ease into a conversation more easily without immediately talking about their emotions or behaviours.

Here is a list of indirect questions that you can ask someone in order to open up a conversation about mental health and how they are feeling. They are also great examples of starting any conversation.

- (Q) What are you up to this evening/afternoon/morning?
- (Q) I was thinking of going for a walk, fancy joining me?

- (Q) What does your perfect holiday look like?
- (Q) Have you seen any good films lately?
- (Q) Have you been working on anything exciting lately?
- (Q) What was the highlight of your week?
- (Q) Are you having a busy time at the moment?
- (Q) What are you doing this weekend?
- (Q) Have you been keeping up with the news recently?
- (Q) I'm going for a coffee, do you want one?
- (Q) Who's your favourite character from a movie/series/book?
- (Q) Have you ever done something like a bungee jump?
- (Q) What piece of advice would your 10-year-old self, give to you right now?
- (Q) When you were growing up, what was your dream job?
- (Q) Who would win in a fight, the Hulk or Superman?
- (Q) What's the most embarrassing thing you did when you were younger?
- (Q) Have you ever met anyone famous?
- (Q) What are you looking forward to this weekend?
- (Q) Have you heard the latest on – news/celebrity/gossip?

- (Q) Where's the most exciting place you've been to?
- (Q) Where do you feel most safe?
- (Q) Would you prefer to be an astronaut or film director?
- (Q) When was the last time you really lost control when laughing?

Guiding A Conversation

Asking one question and getting one answer is a great starting point but a conversation needs to continue. We want to guide the conversation away from harm and negativity. In this section we look at how to deal with answers given to the questions above.

The most important thing to remember is to keep the conversation focused on them. It's fine to talk about your own experiences and own life but don't lose track of the aim of the conversation; which is to talk about their feelings and emotions.

If you get lost in your own words or feel things going in the wrong direction then use one of the following to break up the conversation.

- Pay them a compliment.
- Say something nice about them.

- Let them know that you are both in this together.
- Revert back to an indirect question.
- Talk about their future.

Diverting the conversation is different from guiding a conversation. You should already be aware of the warning signs and risk factors to look out for.

The aim is to ensure the person is safe and is no danger to themselves or others. Should a person look like they are in danger then you need to get them professional help immediately. The seeking help section which is next will show you where to turn for external help.

Here we look at examples of guiding conversations if they fall under the DENP method.

DENP Method:

Dangerous, Emotional, Negative or Positive.

Dangerous

Don't be afraid if the conversation turns into a dangerous situation.

By dangerous I mean if the person is in immediate danger of harm or in danger of harming others. Generally, they would be seeking to self-harm or put themselves in harm's way.

Steps to take:

- Call emergency services.
- Remove all means of self-harm.
- Do not leave them alone.
- Wait for police or ambulance to arrive.
- Let professionals take over.

It can be difficult to resolve a dangerous situation without additional help especially if you're not the type of person to cope with the extreme emotions of another. The removal of any object that can cause the person harm is in the interests of everyone involved.

If you are in a position to help then you might have to move them to a place of safety. This could be their home or somewhere away from other people. It would still make sense to follow the steps above so that professionals can take over from you. It's important to protect your own mental health at the same time.

Emotional

We live in a world where hugging someone can be taken as sexual abuse so it's important to know what you can do and how you can do it.

A person is considered emotional if they are struggling to control their emotions. They may be angry or upset and find it difficult to see beyond their present situation. They might not be in danger of self-harm or harm to others but it doesn't mean that an emotional person may move from emotional to dangerous.

There are some things you can do to help guide a conversation when emotions are running high.

- Be patient.
- Offer to take them to a safe place.
- Do not leave them alone.
- Wait with them until their emotions have calmed down.
- Listen to their needs.
- Ensure that they will be safe.
- Set a time and day to talk again.
- Move them away from other people.
- Use indirect questions (previous section).
- Let them know they are safe.

Unless there is a move to a dangerous level then there is no need to call emergency services purely because someone is emotional. You're in the conversation, whether you started it or not. Aim to not leave a highly emotional person by themselves, they are susceptible to internal and external influences that could lead them into a dangerous situation.

Negative

Conversations may turn negative for many reasons but if you've opened the conversation with someone then it's important to know how to turn negativity into positivity.

The main reason for starting a conversation is to get someone to open up and talk about what's troubling them so there are bound to be negative moments that come up. It doesn't mean that negativity should be shied away from, it shouldn't.

If they need to talk about a traumatic event or what they are feeling then expect some negativity to filter into the conversation. The difference here is recognising when a person is using negativity to feed their own emotions.

To guide a negative conversation back into a positive one you can use some of the following markers to help turn it around.

- Be patient and listen to what they're saying.
- Use direct questions (previous section).
- Use indirect questions (previous section).
- Remind them of something positive in their life.
- Reassure them they are safe.
- Tell them that you're not going anywhere.
- Use future events or activities as a positive marker.
- Talk about your own personal experiences.
- Let them know that professional help is available.

Positive

Just because a conversation goes well and feels good, doesn't mean it should be the end of it. You need to find ways to ensure the conversation continues right then or at another time.

It's important to take any positivity, run with it and then feed it back into the conversation. For example, if they have mentioned something positive about their life then use it as a marker to return to when things are starting to move towards the negative.

Ways of ensuring positivity in a conversation:

- Remind them of their own positive words.
- Use indirect questions (previous section).
- Remind them of something positive in their life.
- If they are happy about something then continue with it.
- Listen to what they say and respond positively.
- Set a time and day when you can talk again.

"It's how we choose to live with time and with ourselves that makes the difference of who we truly are."

Seeking Help

There are different types of help that you can reach out for when someone needs it and it's essential to know when someone needs extra help.

Urgent help is when someone is in immediate danger to themselves or others and the only way to resolve it is by reaching out to professionals. Self-help is where someone is not requiring urgent assistance but can use self-help tools to better their mental health.

Urgent Help

You **MUST** seek urgent help if someone is in immediate danger. First you need to know what immediate danger looks like and what to look out for. You've already started a conversation with them so now you need to look at the deeper signs that something might be wrong.

Things that people might **SAY** when they need immediate help but don't want to ask for it:

- *"It's too late for me."*
- *"I'm in my own endgame now."*
- *"I've already planned for when I'm gone."*
- *"There's nothing left for me in this world."*
- *"I want the world to pay for my sins."*
- *"I don't care about my own life anymore."*
- *"I might cut too deep and see what happens."*
- *"There's nothing you can do to save me."*
- *"No one will come to my funeral."*
- *"No one will miss me."*
- *"I want to take others down with me."*
- *"I can't live like this anymore."*
- *"What's the best way to take my own life?"*

There are many things someone might say when they are at the end of their tether. Mostly, they will talk about how the world doesn't want them, they don't fit in, or no-one will miss them. They will most likely talk about suicide in a very matter-of-fact manner.

Some people might not necessarily talk about things but they will display signs of being in immediate danger.

Here are some examples of what immediate danger might **LOOK** like:

- Active self-harm.
- Selling possessions.
- Putting themselves in harm's way.
- Writing a goodbye letter.
- Saying goodbye to family and friends.
- Actively planning suicide.
- Cutting off communication.
- Isolating themselves from everyone.

"No one has ever become poor by giving."

Anne Frank, Diary Of Anne Frank

Where To Seek Help

A lot of people do not know where to turn to when they are having a mental health crisis or can see that someone else is suffering from one. We sometimes feel afraid to reach out to others for fear of ridicule or being a burden. It's a mindset that need to change.

If we don't reach out then we might miss the opportunity to save someone's life.

If someone is in immediate danger then call the Police.

The police have certain powers to remove someone from the public if they believe they are a danger to themselves or others. It's called a Section 136.

Section 136 is a part of the Mental Health Act that gives powers to the Police to protect someone for up to 24 hours. They can only do so if they believe that they are suffering from a mental illness that requires care or control.

A Section 136 is used when:

- Someone is potentially suffering from a mental disorder.
- It is in the interests of the person's own health or safety.
- It is for the protection of other people around the person.
- Police believe the person needs to be in a place of safety.

A Section 136 can only be extended for a further 12 hours after the statutory 24 hours has passed. The Police will then make all efforts to contact a doctor, nurse or mental health professional when putting someone on a Section 136. They cannot remove a person from their home or any part of their private property under a Section 136.

Most psychiatric hospitals are home to Section 136 rooms where the patient can be seen by a mental health professional. From there a patient can be put on a Section 2, Section 3, or may be discharged from temporary care.

If someone is self-harming or is causing damage to their own body then call an Ambulance.

Paramedics and medical professionals are better placed to be able to fix the injuries of self-harm and get them to a place of safety which is usually the local A&E department of a General Hospital.

Once there, the person will be seen by a mental health professional who will determine the best course of action for them. This might involve being discharged back to home, referred to a community mental health team (CMHT) or be seen by a psychiatrist. In extreme cases, that person might be sectioned under the Mental Health Act and require care within a psychiatric unit.

If you feel that someone requires mental health care but it is not urgent then contact a GP.

Although we say *not urgent*, you should still make it a priority because someone suffering from a mental health crisis is likely to get worse without help. No one we know of has overcome their mental illness without support.

If you know who their doctor or surgery is then you can phone up and make an appointment for them with or without their knowledge. Make sure to say it is urgent. If you don't know who their doctor is then call the non-emergency NHS line on 111 (or relevant service in your country).

A GP is better placed to decide the appropriate course of action for someone with mental health issues. It's important to note that general practitioners are NOT psychiatrists and do not usually diagnose a mental health disorder. They can though offer sleeping aids and mild anti-depressants if they feel they might help in the first instance.

If the GP thinks a patient is in further need of help then they will refer them to a community mental health team or mental health professional, which may include a psychiatrist. A patient has to be referred to a psychiatrist by another medical professional, usually a GP.

There are private therapists and psychiatrists that provide one-to-one sessions but they will cost money. Generally, private therapists charge anything from £50 per session upwards.

Always offer to accompany someone to a GP appointment. Most people are afraid of reaching out and worried about seeing a professional. Some might get an appointment but decide not to go at the last minute. If you offer to go with them, they might feel less alone and more willing to talk. The very act of going to an appointment with someone shows a huge amount of respect for them and what they are feeling.

If you feel that someone would benefit by talking to a mental health professional then use a Helpline.

There are many helplines and services out there with the most famous being The Samaritans. You should encourage them to pick up the phone themselves but if they can't then offer to call first or at least be there with them when they do call.

Here is a list of some of the helplines available in the **United Kingdom**. There are more helplines and organisations listed at the back of the book specifically for the UK.

Samaritans | CALL: 116 123

24 hours a day | 365 days a year.

www.samaritans.org

CALM | CALL: 0800 58 58 58

Campaign Against Living Miserably (CALM)

5pm-midnight | 365 days a year.

www.thecalmzone.net

Hopeline UK | CALL: 0800 068 41 41

Papyrus | Prevention of Young Suicide

www.papyrus-uk.org

SANEline | CALL: 0300 304 7000

SANE | 4:30pm-10:30pm daily.

www.sane.org.uk

Here is a list of the major helplines available in the **United States**.

LIFELINE | CALL: 1-800-273-8255

National Suicide Prevention Helpline | 24/7.

www.suicidepreventionlifeline.org

TrevorLifeline | CALL: 1-866-488-7386

The Trevor Project.

24 hours a day | 365 days a year.

www.thetrevorproject.org

Teen line | CALL: 310-855-4673

6pm-10pm Pacific Time every night.

www.teenlineonline.org

2-1-1 | CALL: **211** (Country-wide)

24 hours a day | 365 days a year.

www.211.org

Sectioning (Mental Health Act)

It's nothing to be afraid of. The Mental Health Act is there to protect individuals from themselves and others.

Being sectioned can be scary and worrying but it can lead to a positive experience. Generally you can be sectioned if you are at risk to yourself or to others, or if your mental health means that you require intensive care for a short or lengthy period of time.

A temporary move to a psychiatric hospital can be incredibly beneficial for those in need. There are different types of sectioning just as there are different types of wards and environments. If someone is sectioned then it's because around-the-clock care is needed to make a person better and keep them safe.

Long gone are the days of Victorian asylums. The mental health wards of today are not unlike any other ward you'll find in a General hospital but are there for long-term use. Most psychiatric wards and hospitals are contained within their own building.

You could be sectioned if:

- You have a suspected mental illness which needs assessment or treatment.
- It is necessary for your health or safety and/or the protection of other people.
- You need to be in hospital to have the assessment or treatment.
- You are unable or unwilling to give your permission to being hospitalised.

If it's not an emergency then a decision is usually made by two doctors and an Approved Mental Health Professional (AMHP). One of the doctors must be specially certified in the assessment or treatment of mental illness, usually a psychiatrist.

If there are concerns about a person's mental health, their own safety, or the safety of others then they can be forced to go to hospital. Most admissions are via an ambulance but can be via the police under the aforementioned Section 136. Most patients within psychiatric units are allowed to leave the hospital for short periods at a time. It is in the form of either escorted or unescorted leave. Escorted leave is usually with a care worker.

Section 2

The Section 2 part of the Mental Health Act is the most commonly used sectioning method. It allows doctors the time to assess the patient which generally leads to a diagnosis and a course of treatment.

A Section 2 is used when:

- Someone is potentially suffering from a mental disorder.
- It is in the interests of the person's own health or safety.
- It is for the protection of other people around the patient.
- A doctor believes they need to be assessed in hospital.

A Section 2 can last up to 28 days from the day of sectioning. It normally ends before 28 days but in some instances the patient may be moved to a Section 3 or become a voluntary patient.

Section 3

Detaining a person under Section 3 of the Mental Health Act is a method of keeping someone in hospital to follow a treatment plan that would not be possible outside of hospital. Psychiatrists and doctor's only use a Section 3 if absolutely necessary and where no alternative can be found.

Most hospital admissions are admitted under a Section 2 for up to 28 days and patients are either discharged at the end of the period or before. Some may go on to become voluntary patients at their own or their doctor's request.

A Section 3 is used when:

- Someone is suffering from a mental disorder that makes it appropriate for them to receive medical treatment in a hospital.
- It is for the protection of the patient or other people around the patient that such treatment should be received.
- The appropriate medical treatment can only be provided in hospital.

A Section 3 can last up to six months from the day of sectioning and can be renewed if required following the end of the first six-month period. The patient will receive a letter detailing their sectioning and the reasons behind it.

Most Section 3's end before the six month period is up and can only be renewed if a patient still requires intensive support. A patient can also be removed from a Section 3 but remain in hospital as a voluntary patient.

A voluntary patient means that instead of going on to a Section 3 from a Section 2, you are able to continue your stay in hospital on a voluntary basis. The main rule about being a voluntary patient is that you must follow the course of recovery laid out by a psychiatrist.

This mostly includes following a course of medication and taking part in therapy or psychology sessions. Should you refuse to follow the course laid out for you then you can be discharged from hospital.

Also, if you fail to return from unescorted leave then your bed on the ward is allocated to a new patient and you lose your right to the bed. This has been common from 2019 due to the lack of mental health beds available in NHS facilities.

There are other section types available but the ones shown in this book are the most commonplace.

Self Help

The most popular self-help tools are known as coping strategies and they are detailed in the coping strategies section of this book. This section deals with how you can help another person to help themselves.

They say that if you have knowledge then you should share that knowledge freely to others so that it can help them. There are many different methods of self-help which involve everything from walking to regular visits. We take a look at some of them below.

First things you should do:

- Don't wait to be asked, offer and ask first.
- Be specific with how you can assist.
- Don't give up, be persistent.

There is a school of thought that claims we should not ask someone; "*How can I help*?" The theory behind it is that if you are asking someone if they need help then you are already assuming they are helpless.

I disagree, it only works that way in professional business conversations where someone might take offence to you if you offer help in their business. In personal relations, fire away! There's nothing wrong with asking someone if they need help.

Self-help examples:

- Go for a morning or evening walk.
- Create a routine.
- Do something that challenges them like a quiz.
- Removing the phrase 'I should' from their vocabulary.

- Take a nap when they feel tired during the day.
- Gain new knowledge in history or geography.
- Get involved in a new hobby.
- Rearrange items in the bedroom.
- Read an informative book or website.
- Declutter by giving some older items to charity.
- Turn off the internet connection for at least one hour.
- Do a jigsaw puzzle.
- Listen to an audiobook.
- Start a journal either in a diary or as a blog.
- Listen to some feel-good music.
- Write down a list of things you are grateful for.
- Give to a food bank.
- Help out at a local charity shop or service.
- Mute toxic accounts on social media.
- Get rid of the bathroom scale!
- Dance to your favourite song in any style you wish.
- Do some stretching exercises.
- Practice Yoga or Tai-Chi.
- Go to bed earlier than usual.
- Join a local community group.
- Shadow-punch to remove stress.
- Take a long hot bath or shower.
- Bake something you've never baked before.

- Cook a meal you wouldn't normally have.
- Buy or pick some flowers.
- Self-massage your muscles.
- Go to a comedy club or evening.
- Revisit some favourite childhood films or books.
- Style your hair differently.
- Watch funny YouTube videos.
- Avoid loud noises and large crowds.
- Light some incense.
- Make yourself a fancy coffee or hot chocolate.

A lot of self-help ideas, as with coping strategies, take time to practice and get right. Don't give up, utilising self-help methods can go a long way to help with negative thoughts and emotions.

"You wouldn't be able to lift the heavy weights without having practised with the lighter ones first."

Coping Strategies

There is the well-known adage that mental health disorders are never fully cured; only managed. The same tools can be provided for those at risk of suicide. By helping someone to help themselves, they stand a better chance at life. This coping strategies sections is full of relevant, helpful, and life-changing information.

Use them! Push others to use them!

The tools and exercises provided here can help you feel happier, more productive, increase confidence/self-esteem, and help you move towards understanding and using self-compassion

Distraction

Distraction or avoidance is an important coping strategy because it can immediately help with overwhelming feelings and emotions. Distraction techniques use both mental and physical processes to ensure you have a complete skill set.

It's also a great idea to practice all coping strategies and self-help tools at times when you don't feel the need for them. This way you can practice them well in preparation and see what works best for you. As with all self-help tools and coping mechanisms, you should practice them over and over until such time that they become a natural part of your thought processes.

It takes time, so try not to worry if you can't get it right straight away.

Positive Memory

Think of a place either imagined or real that you find safe, relaxing or beautiful. If you don't have a positive memory or good experience that you can draw upon then you can create one.

It doesn't always mean physically going out and seeking a perfectly happy experience, it never normally happens that way. Instead, create a perfect place in your head that you can retreat to.

Imagine you are the director of a video playing in your mind. You have the power of adding elements to create a perfect scene that can make you happy and content.

Some positive memory ideas:

- Focus on an actual positive memory.
- A place in the world you want to travel to.
- Imagine a perfect waterfall.

- Imagine a wondrous jungle or landscape.
- People who are a positive influence.
- Happy moments with friends or by yourself.
- Aromas that make you happy such as fresh bread or hot chocolate.
- Remember a happy holiday you went on.
- Think back to a concert or theatre show that made you happy.
- Use taste to access positive memories.

Really focus your mind on a positive image. Notice all the small details and intricacies that only you can see. The aim is to replace negative emotions and thoughts with positive ones that can overpower them.

When you feel your thoughts drifting to bad experiences or memories then force that positive image back into your mind. You might then feel the negative emotions drain out of you like a cube of ice on a barbecue!

Alternative Emotion

It doesn't mean finding an alternative to emotion because there is no alternative. Emotions are what make us who we are and it's only right to embrace them. It's how we use emotion that makes the difference. Alternating emotions to bring yourself back into the moment is a psychological tool that has been used for decades.

It's a skill whereby you choose the opposite action or emotion to how you're feeling. It means to deliberately seek a different emotional state of being.

It's not obvious emotions either, for example if you're feeling sad (not depressed, there is a difference!) then you could do something that scares you to swap sadness for fear. All emotions are positive in some way because they allow us to function within a human society.

Fear is important to our state of well-being and so is happiness. Distracting yourself with a different emotion is one way to control any negativity that may arise.

On the next page are some things you can do when you find yourself in an overwhelming emotional state.

- Read a joke book or joke website.
- Watch a comedy film or TV series.
- Take part in an online quiz (it focuses your attention).
- Watch a scary movie.
- Listen to uplifting music.
- Read a life-affirming book.
- Write a happy note for yourself to find later.
- Go outside for some fresh air to help calm you.
- Try a bit of online shopping therapy.

- Switch off the internet.
- Write down your thoughts onto paper or a blog.
- Learn new things from educational YouTube videos.
- Make your favourite drink.

You might not have a joke book or have access to the internet but you might have access to a comedy film on DVD. It doesn't matter how you distract yourself, the list above is interchangeable, what matters is that you DO distract yourself with a different emotion.

Utilising alternative emotions can work very well for those who are prone to anger or heavy waves of sadness. Practice them even when you're not feeling overwhelmed because then you'll already know how to distract yourself when things do get on top of you.

Physical Distraction

This works well with grounding techniques in the next section as it is the art of physically removing yourself from a situation where you might be losing control. You could find yourself having a severe blast of anxiety or find it difficult to cope with an overpowering emotion.

By physically distracting yourself, you are focusing your emotions and thoughts on a positive action. This engages the mind with a different focus and can be extremely beneficial.

Physical distraction doesn't have to be exercise and fitness routines – although it does help – it could be as simple as doing something with your hands.

Here are some ideas and examples of physical distraction:

- Play a sport you enjoy.
- Go to the gym and use your favourite machines.
- Take a walk to a local park or beach.
- Make something from scratch such as a DVD shelf.
- Start painting or drawing.
- Get on top of that housework you've been putting off.
- Engage in or find a hobby.
- Do some simple body-weight exercises.
- Take a long shower.
- Tense and flex your fingers to relieve tension.
- Focus on breathing techniques.
- Self-massage.
- Dust off the Nintendo Wii and play Wii Sports!
- Play an instrument.

- Use your hands to tap the beat of your favourite song.
- Play a game like snooker or darts.

Physical distraction doesn't have to be hard but the more you practice, the easier it will become.

"Even the smallest act of kindness can make a big difference."

Grounding

Grounding techniques are used to bring yourself back into the present moment. It's not the same as '*earthing*' which is reconnecting yourself to nature, sometimes referred to as grounding.

Grounding can be a powerful tool to have at your disposal when you find yourself becoming disconnected from reality. It works by reconnecting your senses to the present to give you back control and safety.

You might think that some of the skills shown in this coping strategies section seem a little mundane and obvious. Not all techniques work for every individual, you should find what works for you and run with it. If it doesn't work for you after practice then go and try something else. You might be surprised what works and what doesn't.

Grounding can help regain focus, keep you calm, overcome anxiety and decrease stress. Grounding techniques can provide you with the skills to help break the cycle.

Mental Grounding

Describe your current surroundings

Literally talk about the present!

When describing your surroundings, focus on the colours, shapes, smells, sounds and anything else you notice or that stands out to you. Try to follow a logical line of self-questioning and description.

For example:

- Where are you sitting?
- What are you sitting on?
- What's right in front of you?

- What type of room are you in?
- What colour are the walls?
- Is there any noise from outside?
- Is there an aroma in the air?
- What objects are around you?
- What do the objects look like?
- Use all senses to describe your surroundings.

Describe your surroundings in as much detail as possible to better focus your mind. The more detail you can provide yourself, no matter how mundane, the quicker you will be able to regain control of your thoughts and ground yourself in the present.

Explain what you are currently doing

There is a difference between describing your surroundings and explaining what you are doing. When describing what you are currently doing, there might not be any physical thing to describe so you have to focus on your actions and not your surroundings.

Some examples:

- Are you walking or sitting?
- What does it feel like?
- What are you doing right now?

- Are your muscles hurting?
- Do you have any aches?
- What are you doing with your hands?
- Can you see each part of your body?
- Are you doing something important?
- Can you describe what you are physically feeling?

It's easy to zone-out and detach from reality when your thoughts wander off in all kinds of negative directions. By describing what you are doing, you are mentally bringing yourself back into the present moment and refocusing your attention to your actions and what is going on around you.

Have fun with mental grounding

Maybe it's not appropriate to describe your surroundings or what you are doing but there are things you can do in your own head to bring you back into the present moment.

Do you like films? Music? Books? Gardening? Kung-Fu!? You can incorporate whatever you enjoy doing into a mental grounding technique. Think of it as your own private mental health quiz in your head.

On the following page are some things you can do based around what you might enjoy. Adapt the items in the list for something you prefer or think you can answer.

- Name an actor/actress and then 10 films they have appeared in.
- Name a band and all their album titles.
- Name some animals in alphabetical order.
- Think of your favourite film and then name all the actors.
- Think of an author and name all of their books.
- Try and name all the types of plants in your garden.
- Come up with alternative titles to films, books or songs.
- Name the current top 10 in the music charts.
- Name as many films/albums/books that are coming out this year.
- Think of a sport and name winning teams/individuals by year.
- Think about the last time you completed a video game and the steps you took to get to the end.
- Think of all the buttons used when playing a game.
- Name famous mountains or lakes.

Physical Grounding

There are a lot of ways that you can physically ground yourself. It's a way of forcing yourself back into the present to ensure that negative thoughts and emotions don't carry you away.

Grounding is important because it stops you from becoming further dissociated from reality. Being detached from the present moment can lead to higher anxiety, depression, a feeling of hopelessness and paranoia.

Physically grounding yourself can sometimes generate higher levels of concentration.

Here are some examples of what physical grounding can look like.

- Sit or stand more upright.
- Touch and describe objects around you.
- Push your feet into the floor and really feel it.
- Eat a food with a strong taste.
- Put your hands in a sink of cold water.
- Put your face into a bowl of cold water.
- Hold a cup of tea and feel its warmth.
- Stretch the part of you that feels tense.

- Rotate your shoulders to relax your shoulders.
- Turn your head to each side and stretch your neck out.
- Use muscle relaxation (next section).
- Use breathing techniques (next section).
- Aim to physically feel the air around you.
- Run your fingers along a wall or tree.
- Push your index finger and thumb together.
- Use your thumb and fingers to squeeze the opposite palm.
- Make fists with your hands then relax them.
- Use any combination of stretches that make you feel good.
- Rub your thighs to release tension.
- Flip off your shoe and rub your feet.
- Lift your hands high above your head and hold until tired.

When practicing physical grounding, ensure to be aware of how it feels. Notice the details and describe every element of it; the colour, texture, material, flavour, and feel of it. Notice temperature, surfaces, the feeling of your own body and the objects that you touch.

Physical grounding can also lead to you discovering more about yourself, your own body and the benefits it can bring to your mental health.

Soothing Grounding

Soothing is often related to having a '*Soothe Box*' where people keep small items that make them happy. It's a commonly used psychological tool akin to having a happy place to retreat to. A soothe box can contain personal artefacts that bring you peace, make you happy and ground you in the present moment.

Instead of a soothe box, you can carry small items of personal importance that you can use as reminder of positive memories or times. Either way can work just as well.

When we talk about soothing in grounding, it's not too dissimilar from using positive memory techniques. Both mean to focus on something positive but soothing is not just mental, it can be physical as well.

Some examples of soothing grounding techniques:

- Think of people who are a positive influence.
- Use positive imagery to distract and ground you (previous section).
- Carry a photo or reminder of a person you love.
- Think of positive future events or dates.
- Remind yourself it's okay to relax.

- Use a 'soothe box' to open in times of need.
- Keep something special or sentimental on your person.
- Write yourself positive notes to randomly hide around the house.
- Keep a marble in your pocket and hold it when you feel overwhelmed.
- Buy a gemstone to funnel your positivity in to.
- Use a piece of fabric to remind you of something positive.
- Describe your soothing object in as much detail as you can.

It can also be a good idea to write down or print any of the distraction or grounding techniques shown in this book.

Cut out a small A6 piece of card that you can leave somewhere safe, the back of a cereal box will do. When you need to use the techniques to help focus then you can consult the card at any time. Keep it on your person if you're likely to experience negative emotions whilst outside the house.

"You have already been given the tools for your own survival."

Relaxation

Relaxation sounds easy but is it really?

If you're suffering from mental health issues or negative thoughts, it can be difficult to relax at any time of the day or night. Relaxation methods can be both mental and physical, there is no rule as to what makes one person relax and not another.

You might need to relax if you are:

- Overthinking.
- Worrying too much.
- Stressed.
- Having negative thoughts.
- Have a high heart rate.
- High blood pressure.
- Headaches.
- Aches and pains.
- Feeling hopeless.
- Feeling tired or worn out.
- Being physically exhausted.

Do not confuse relaxation with laziness.

Laziness means to be unwilling to work or use energy.

Relaxation means to be free of anxiety and tension.

It's not always possible to avoid stress due to the way in which we might live our lives but stress can be managed. We manage stress primarily through relaxation.

When our bodies relax, we are increasing the flow of blood which enables us to lower our heart rates and reduce blood pressure. Doing so relieves tension. It can help with disbanding negative thoughts and give us a fresh outlook on a situation.

Stress is a physical reaction that plays on mental processes. By understanding and using some of the tools in the following sections, you will be able to relax at any time of the day and anywhere.

Mindfulness

You might have heard of mindfulness being touted as part of the ritual of meditation. Although similar, it's not quite the same but is sometimes known as mindful meditation. It is potentially the greatest psychological tool that you can arm yourself with.

Mindfulness means to ground yourself and your thoughts in the present moment. Too often we let our thoughts drift to bad memories of the past or unwarranted fears of the future. We rarely focus entirely on the present moment. This is what the art of mindfulness can help us with.

Mindfulness is found in all walks of life and is being taught all over the world. There are mindfulness mentors, therapists, retreat days, groups, resources, educational books and guides all over the place and there's particularly good reason for it; mindfulness works.

It does mean that there are a million and one ways to practice mindfulness and it's mostly due to how an individual lives their life and the environment around them.

Here we look at some of the more popular methods and exercises of mindfulness. As always, mindfulness, just like any self-help tool or coping strategy, takes practice.

You wouldn't be able to play the first violin in an orchestra without having started as a beginner somewhere along the line.

Water For Mindfulness

Run your hands under water

It sounds simple and it is. If you're lucky enough to have a waterfall nearby then you're probably already making the most of it. If not and that goes for most of us then the simple exercise of putting your hands under a running tap can help.

Go for either cold or warm water, whichever you prefer. As you move your hands through the water, notice the way it flows over and between your hands.

Take a shower

We all should be showering at least once a day to protect our health and hygiene, so the very act of taking a shower is embedded into our daily lives and routine.

Next time you take a shower, really listen to the sound of the water falling around you and focus on the way it feels. Even try using a different soap with different aromas to focus your senses.

Sip a glass of water

Grab a glass or cup of water and sip at it very slowly. Sense the water touch your lips and notice the way it feels against your skin. Taking your time to practice exercises like this can reap huge benefits for a more positive mental health. You could also try and drink from the tap instead of using a glass.

Place your hands in a bowl of water

Makes sure the water's not too cold or too hot, you want it to feel comfortable and gentle on the skin. Lower your hands in and feel the water surround your fingers before completely submerging your hands. Move your hands around in the water to feel different sensations. You can also add a few drops of tea tree oil or similar into the bowl for added sensations.

Submerge your face in water

This is one of the most beneficial mindfulness exercises that utilises water. It's also a fantastic grounding technique that can be practised by anyone. Some people find it easier to hold their nose when submerging their head in the water and that's more than fine, whatever works for you.

Use cold water! Cold water constricts blood vessels and can help reduce any swelling or inflammation you may have. It also numbs nerve endings and can bring immediate relief to pain.

Food For Mindfulness

The beauty of using food for mindfulness is that you can practice it every time you sit down for a meal or grab a bite to eat.

For some people it works better if you make your favourite dinner or consume your favourite food. Using food for mindfulness might not be possible for some people due to any manner of eating disorders or other reasons, so don't feel that you have to try something if it doesn't feel right for you.

Here are some ideas for using food with mindfulness:

- Notice the texture.
- Take time to taste your food.
- Describe the taste.
- Notice the sound when you chew.
- Describe the colours.
- What does the food feel like in your hands?
- What does the food feel like in your mouth?
- Think about where the food has come from.
- Describe how it makes you feel.

We're constantly being told what to eat by the media, government, friends and gossip sites but you don't have to listen to them. If you're really struggling and someone's telling you to eat more healthily then it's not really going to help matters.

There is an unwritten rule in psychology that it doesn't matter what you eat as long as you are eating so don't be afraid to eat a bit of junk food every now and again. You could set aside a day each week to really enjoy your favourite guilty pleasure.

"It's not for the world to accept us, we have to accept ourselves first."

Nature For Mindfulness

We're not all lucky enough to live beside a roaming countryside or mountain range but there is nature around you, it's just a case of finding it. You can adapt your surroundings to fit in with using nature for mindfulness.

Describe the view from your window

Nature isn't necessarily blue seas and green trees, there is nature to be found in cities and populated areas as well. Sit or stand next to your window and look out at the view. Notice the weather and how it makes you feel. Look for trees, plants or animals and describe what they look like. Use colours, sensations, smells and movements to describe them in more detail.

Imagine using the window as a frame to take a snapshot of the world beyond the glass. Imagine that the view from your window is a painting and that you are describing what you see to someone over the phone.

Notice the greenery on a walk to town

Even in a city, there will be a hanging basket on a shop door frame or trees lining a road. Even the smallest piece of nature can work. Make sure to notice as much as possible. Slow down if need be, there's no reason to storm into town as fast as you can. Take time to feel the breeze, sunlight, or rain on your face. Notice the way a tree sways in the wind and watch its leaves move in unique ways.

Purchase some flowers or a plant

For a small price, you can get hold of a small bunch of flowers, better yet a large plant. Once you get home, take the time to tidy up the stems or leaves, wash everything down gently and then put them into a nice vase or jug of water. Place them somewhere noticeable and enjoy them. If you start to feel disconnected from reality then describe the flowers in detail, taking the time to notice every little thing about them.

If you can't afford to purchase flowers and can access the countryside or forest park then go foraging! Pick some wildflowers or blades of a tall grass and take them home.

Spend more time with your pet or at a petting zoo

If you have a pet then spend more time with them, be compassionate and caring and use the time you have to achieve a positive outcome. Pets can provide us with happiness and laughter, they can be there for you when others might not be able to. If you don't have a pet then there are petting zoos in most cities where you can go to spend some time with animals. You might find it to be an extremely therapeutic experience.

If you don't have a pet or access to a petting zoo then you could pay a visit to a local farm and see if you can help out for a bit. It's always best to phone ahead. Don't be afraid of getting in contact with a farm, most farmers will welcome a bit of assistance at any time of the year.

Do some gardening

If you have a garden then you will most likely have a bedding area or plant pots. Gardening can involve so many different elements such as weeding, creating new flowerbeds, vegetable patches, tidying up or mowing the grass. Gardening is very repetitive which is perfect for keeping your mind focused on the present and allows you to be creative with your landscaping.

If you don't have a garden then you can apply for an allotment or see if you can help a neighbour with theirs. You could also ask an older person if they need help maintaining their own garden. You never know, you might even make a new friend out of it.

Spend time at a beach or waterfall

Head to a local beach or waterfall. It doesn't have to be anything extravagant, we're not always blessed with living next to 100-metre waterfalls but even a small stream that trickles under a bridge will do. Notice the sounds, the smells and the movement of the water. Relax your mind and let the power of water metaphorically flow over you.

If you don't have access to a beach or waterfall then there are other ways around it. You can find an image online, watch a film that has a beach or waterfall in or even use meditation. Sit down, close your eyes and simply imagine a perfect waterfall or shoreline and then use all your senses to describe it.

Go forest bathing!

Forest bathing is a real thing! It's also known as forest therapy and is a more recent tool to allow people from the cities to reconnect with nature. Visit a local forest or country park and sit down against a tree. Relax yourself and then engage all of your senses with the surroundings.

Notice the movement of the leaves, the sound of the wind coming through the trees, the aroma of the land and the sunlight breaking through the canopy. Become indulgent with your surroundings and find peace with yourself, if just for a moment.

Take a packed-lunch and your favourite drink to extend the experience. If you don't live near a forest or country park then use your local inner-city park or garden to reconnect with nature.

Some of the benefits of forest bathing include:

- Connecting to nature through all the senses.
- Feeling alive with the peace of the forest.
- Being fully aware of the beauty of nature.
- The earthly feeling that being in nature brings.
- A new-found care and compassion for nature.

If you don't have access to natural features in any way then you can still practice mindfulness by using photographs. They can be physical or online photos, it doesn't matter which.

Find an image that you find striking or pleasurable and describe it in detail. Take the time to enjoy the colours, the shadows and the feeling of it. Imagine yourself being there.

Imagination is important because it is the faculty of the soul.

Breathing Exercises

We all do it but there are ways of breathing that can reduce stress, help with negative thought and relax our physical bodies. When your body becomes stressed, you breathe in more than you breathe out. This keeps your body on high-alert. Breathing slowly and deeply can provide a simple way to calm the body.

The simple process of just focusing on your breathing can help enormously. It's not surprising at all that breathing exercises are among the most popular stress and anxiety self-help tools available.

When we talk about breathing exercises we're not talking about incidental breathing which is the kind you need to do to survive. We're talking about deep and focused breathing. It's about being aware of your own body, how it works and how you can use it to fight off negative thought and emotion.

The benefits of deep breathing include lower stress, increased concentration, lower blood pressure and improved health, both physically and mentally. Like every self-help tool and coping strategy, it requires practice and the more you practice the easier it will become.

Deep Breathing Method 1

Also known as belly breathing, abdominal breathing or diaphragmatic breathing.

Follow each of these steps:

- Place your hands on your rib cage.
- Focus on taking 10 slow and deep breaths.
- When you breathe in, feel your ribs expand.
- Focus on 360-degree expansion of the upper body.
- Your belly shouldn't be the only thing that moves.

Feel the expansion of the rib cage with every breath. You can place your thumb on your lower ribs with your fingers resting underneath on your belly. When you focus on a deep breath, you should feel your fingers move further outwards than your thumbs.

Deep breathing can even improve back and neck pain because you're allowing your lungs to fill up rather than using shallow breathing. Filling your lungs means that your rib cage will expand which can help with any aches or pains.

Deep Breathing Method 2

Deep breathing can stop air from remaining in your lungs too long. Having trapped air can cause you to breathe in more quickly and not exhale the old air.

- Push your elbows comfortably back behind you.
- This allows your chest to expand easier.
- Inhale deeply to fill your lungs.
- Hold your breath as you count to 5.
- Breathe out in a slow and controlled manner.

There is a misconception that you have to breathe in through your nose and out through mouth. If you don't feel comfortable breathing in through your nose then you don't have to do it that way, it's not a rule. Whatever feels comfortable for you is the **BEST** way of doing it.

When exhaling or holding your breath you may feel dizzy so remember to be mindful of your surroundings and practice breathing exercises in safety. Sitting on the bed or a comfortable chair can be good starting points.

Breathe out MORE than you breathe in

When your body is stressed or anxious then you breathe in more than you do when you are calm. Reverse the process by breathing out more than you breathe in.

- Breathe in for 1 beat then out for 1-2
- Breathe in for 1 beat then out for 1-2 then REST
- Breathe in for 1 beat then out for 1-2 then RELAX

You don't need to breathe in straight after you breathe out.

Say the letters out loud between breaths because you're always breathing out when you talk.

- R.E.S.T (4 beats)
- R.E.L.A.X. (5 beats)

A beat is as long or as short as you feel comfortable with. It could be two seconds or five, you know your own body better than anyone else.

Let your body guide you.

Muscle Relaxation

Muscle relaxation is also known as Progressive Muscle Relaxation (PMR). It is a powerful physical and mental coping strategy to help control stress and anxiety.

When your body is wound-up and anxious it can feel tense and tight. These pains and stresses can be alleviated by using PMR. There are many short ways to practice it along with dedicated PMR programmes. The trick is to tense a certain muscle group then suddenly release the tension and feel the muscle relax.

If you have any pains in a certain area then you don't have to force yourself to tense that muscle.

Muscle relaxation can help lower stress, help with sleeping and improve both physical and mental health. It's also a fantastic mindfulness tool that directs attention to parts of our body we might not normally interact with. This allows us to understand and better appreciate our physical self.

Full Body Muscle Relaxation

There are many methods of muscle relaxation that you could use. There's no right or wrong way of doing it. You can practice sitting or standing, whichever you find more comfortable.

- Begin by calming the body with Deep Breathing (previous section).
- Aim to tense each muscle for 10 seconds before suddenly relaxing.
- Begin with the forehead then neck and shoulders.

- Move down to the chest, abdomen then thighs.
- Then the leg muscles and feet to complete it.

Aim to go through every single muscle and muscle group from the top down. Remember not to strain and if it aches then move onto the next muscle group. Think of it as a body check-up protocol! Check each section of your muscular structure to see if it's in working order.

Quick & Easy Fixes

Sometimes you might wish to alleviate the tension quicker than normal and have no time for a full body relaxation session. Which is where quick and easy fixes come in.

Any of the following can be practiced anywhere and at any time you feel tension rising in your body. They really are quick and easy to do and can help immeasurably.

- Lift your shoulders high to your chin.
- Turn your head to the side (15 seconds each side).
- Outstretch your arms and tense every arm muscle.
- Make fists and then drop them to relax.
- Tense your butt muscles.
- Stand on tiptoes for 30 secs or longer then drop.
- Make fists with your toes.
- Lift your arms up above your shoulders and hold for 30 seconds.

Remember to abruptly relax after 30 seconds. If you still feel tense then go again or try a muscle group that works better for you. If you find that muscle relaxation is helpful then you could incorporate it into a longer-term exercise goal. It could include going to the gym, practising Yoga or Tai-Chi.

Self-Massage

Massaging your own muscles is not always linked with Progressive Muscle Relaxation but it can be a fantastic way to release muscle tension. If you've ever rubbed your shoulders when you feel tense then you know just how good and relaxing it can be.

Examples of self-massage:

- Squeeze each arm up to the shoulders.
- Using both hands, gently massage your neck.
- Sit down and knead the soles of your feet.
- When sitting, squeeze and massage your calves.
- Stand up and massage your lower back.

If it hurts to push a certain muscle group then take it easy on that section. You can self-massage most places on your body with ease but there are self-massaging devices on the market at various price-levels. If you're lucky enough to have a partner who doesn't mind giving massages then take them up on the offer!

Myths Debunked

There are so many misconceptions surrounding mental health and suicide. Read about some of the myths below along with what the facts really are.

MYTH: When breathing deeply you have to breathe in through your nose and out through your mouth.

FACT: It doesn't matter if you breathe in through your fish gills! If you find it more comfortable breathing in and out through your mouth then it is right for you.

MYTH: Only teenage girls self-harm.

FACT: Self-harm is not limited to a certain sex or age and can affect anyone at any time in their lives.

MYTH: People who self-harm belong to the Goth or Metal crowds.

FACT: Self-harm does not discriminate against certain music choices.

MYTH: Mental health issues don't affect that many people.

FACT: An estimated 25% of all people will be affected by mental health issues at some point in their lives. 1 in 4 is a lot.

MYTH: People with mental health problems are violent and unpredictable.

FACT: Those who suffer from mental health issues are more likely to have been a victim of violence than an aggressor.

MYTH: Being mentally ill is a sign of weakness.

FACT: Being physically injured or ill is not a sign of weakness nor is being mentally ill. Those who learn to manage their mental illness are actually incredibly strong and brave.

MYTH: Mental health statistics are exaggerated for government purposes.

FACT: If that was true then mental health would be better funded. Most mental health stats come from official and recognised sources such as the World Health Organisation, Center for Disease Control, National Health Service and the Office of National Statistics.

MYTH: People with schizophrenia are violent psychopaths.

FACT: You've probably been watching too many horror films. Violence is NOT a symptom of schizophrenia.

MYTH: People with DID, BPD or schizophrenia have split personalities.

FACT: It is biologically impossible for someone to split their personalities. DID sufferers can develop different personality **types** but it is not the same as having split personalities.

MYTH: Eating disorders only affect females.

FACT: Eating disorders do not discriminate against sex. Every gender, race and age group are susceptible to developing an eating disorder.

MYTH: People fake mental illness to get sympathy.

FACT: Mental illness can be upsetting, stressful and painful to live with. It would be extremely rare for someone to fake a mental illness.

MYTH: People who self-harm only want attention.

FACT: Self harm can be a cause OR consequence of mental health. To physically damage your own body is a sign of needing help. Using self-harm to get attention is in itself displaying some form of mental issue.

MYTH: Depression only happens after a traumatic event.

FACT: Depression can affect anyone at any time for any reason. There is no singular cause for depression.

MYTH: Suicide is an easy way out.

FACT: Suicide is never normally an impulsive act, it is usually thought about and planned beforehand. It is the most damaging consequence of mental illness. What a suicidal person goes through is not easy in any way.

MYTH: People who talk about suicide will not do it themselves.

FACT: The very act of talking about suicide can be a major warning sign of suicide itself. They might be talking about it as a way to get attention to the fact that they need help.

MYTH: Suicidal people want to die.

FACT: Generally if someone is thinking about suicide it's because they want a different life to the one they have, they don't necessarily want to die. Many factors lead to the belief that it is the only option when it is not.

MYTH: If someone is suicidal once then they will always be suicidal.

FACT: There may be some crossover of suicidal thought but with the right help, people can overcome or maintain the underlying issues that originally led to them becoming suicidal.

MYTH: Talking about suicide is bad.

FACT: Being open about suicide is one way to get others talking about their feelings. Talking about suicide is never bad if spoken about in a constructive manner.

MYTH: People are only suicidal if they have mental health issues.

FACT: There might be an underlying issue with some but suicidal ideation is something that can happen to anyone for any reason regardless of who they are or where they come from.

MYTH: Suicide is a spontaneous act.

FACT: Suicide is usually thought about and planned beforehand. Rarely is it an instinctive action that someone will take. However, it's still important to know the warning signs.

MYTH: You shouldn't ask someone if they're thinking of suicide.

FACT: If you're talking to someone about their mental health and they seem extremely negative or suffering from depression then it's okay to ask them if they are planning to hurt themselves. Even if they don't respond positively then you have opened the doorway to a more meaningful conversation.

Suicide Prevention Life Plan

What is it?

A life plan is a roadmap for your life that helps you find what is important to you. It helps focus your attention on moving towards your desired life.

Most people make the mistake of sticking to a life plan exactly as it's written but you need to be able to adapt to changes. When something goes wrong or when life takes a different turn, your life plan might go out of the window but it doesn't have to be a permanent change,

Think of your life plan as a guide that allows change when and where necessary. It's something to fall back on when you're feeling low or lost and something to use to bring you back into the present in the same way that grounding techniques do.

It is your personal guide to how you live, what is important to you and what you need to do to reach certain goals in life.

A suicide prevention life plan is exactly that! It's a life plan written in such a way that you can reach out to it when needed to put you back on the right track. It helps with mental health issues, negative emotions and negative thoughts.

In this section, you're going to learn how to write a suicide prevention life plan so that you can use it to help others or help yourself.

Before you say; "*I can't write*" or "*it sounds too hard*", take a look at what you might already be doing in your day-to-day routine.

Do you:

- Text friends?
- Message on social media?
- Post on Facebook?
- Tweet to others?
- Comment on social media?
- Write a blog?
- Use a search engine?
- Write Birthday cards?

If you do at least one of the above then you **CAN** write your life plan.

Your life plan doesn't have to be the next literary marvel, nor does it have to be comprehensible to others. If you can understand what you've written then that's all you need.

It's important to have a suicide prevention life plan because it allows you to take control of your life and your future. Even if we account for various changes in your life, you can still look back at your life plan for some form of guidance, to at least put you back on the right track.

A suicide prevention life plan might look a little different from a generalised life plan. It's designed to keep you thinking about how you live your life and not how to end it.

Step 1: Interview Yourself

Step one is usually the self-assessment stage but I think that sounds too formal so I've changed it to a self-interview. This is done in two stages.

The **first stage** is interviewing yourself about your life **now**.

The **second stage** is interviewing yourself in the **future**.

It will all make sense in a moment!

Stage One

Stage one is where you interview yourself from another's perspective. The idea behind it is to ask yourself questions and then answer them truthfully about your life in the present.

You could use any of the following as a way to interview yourself:

- An author writing a book about you.
- Being interviewed for a documentary.
- On stage in front of an audience.
- A reporter writing an article about you.
- An archivist adding your information to a database.
- A friend asking questions about your life.

There are many questions that you can ask yourself and they might be individual to you. I've listed some here as a guide you can use to work from or adapt. The aim of these questions is to find out about your life in the present.

Examples of questions you can ask yourself in a self-interview:

- Where do you want to be in ten years' time?
- What are you grateful for in your life?
- What do you love most in the world?
- Who do you love most in the world?
- Why do you self-harm?
- Do you worry too much about what others think?
- What does the future look like to you?
- What would you do if you wasn't afraid of anything?
- What would you do if today was your last day?

- Is your social network mostly negative or positive?
- Are you involved in any toxic friendships or relationships?
- Are your family members caring towards you?
- Do you think that your family is good for your mental health?
- Is your physical health up to a good enough standard?
- Do you eat healthily?
- Are you giving enough time to the people you most care about?
- Do you care too much about how you look?
- Do you appreciate that your soul is worth more than your body?
- Is there anything you are running away from?
- Where do your fears come from?
- What would be your biggest regret if you were to die tomorrow?
- What are the core values that you live by?
- What contribution to the world will you leave behind?
- If money was no object, where in the world would you want to visit?
- Who inspires you the most?
- What inspires you the most?

- Who is the person who most makes you happy in the world?
- What does success look like to you?
- What are your hopes for the future?
- What are your dreams for the future?
- What does your perfect day look like?
- What is the biggest failure in your life?
- What is the biggest success you've had in your life?
- What would change the most about your life?
- What are you afraid of the most?
- Are you happy where you live right now?
- What opportunities are you looking for right now?
- How would you describe yourself?
- What will you do differently after reading this book?

Stage Two

This is where you interview yourself in the future but don't worry, it's easier than you think. You just have to use a little imagination!

Imagine you are able to time-travel and you travel to visit your future self a few decades from now. You are able to ask your future self, questions about what they have achieved and their experiences in life.

The aim here is to find out what kind of goals you can set in the present that will positively affect you in the future. You can use the same questions above to gauge what might be different but there's also a whole new list of questions you can use to explore your future.

Examples of questions you can ask yourself in the future:

- Is there another person I can interview about your life?
- What is one thing you were afraid of but overcame?
- What is the one thing you thought you would never do but did it?
- What has been your greatest success?
- Where have you lived and who have you lived with?
- Have you worked hard to get to where you are?
- What is most important to you now?
- Who are the people that are most important to you?
- What are your core values?
- What habits do you have now that you didn't have before?
- Are you aware of how you fit into the world?
- How do you handle stressful situations?
- What is your home environment like?
- What are your friends like?
- What does a typical day look like?
- What can others remember you for?
- What is the greatest achievement of your life?

- Did your fears about life ever materialise?
- How has your journey through life panned out?
- Did you manage to live out some of your dreams?
- What was the most important thing you learned in life?
- What advice would you give your past self?
- Is there something you're still holding on to?
- What changed in your life that you least expected to?
- What was the biggest change that positively influenced you?
- Have you lived the best life possible?
- What do you wish you had done but never did?
- What were the lottery numbers two decades earlier?

The last one was light-hearted but if you managed to time travel then it probably would be the first thing to find out!

Asking yourself questions is one way to gauge how your life is currently doing and what you might need to do to make any positive changes. The next step is turning those answers into priorities.

At the end of the life plan section I have included an example of what a life plan might look like so you can see how to fit all these different elements together to create a positive plan for the present and the future.

Step 2: Setting Priorities

From the questions you've asked yourself in Step 1, you've probably already realised that there are some things more important to you than others. No life plan will be the same so just because someone says a particular thing is a priority in their life doesn't mean it should or could be in yours.

The interesting and obvious thing about priorities is that they change over time. Priorities as a 20-year-old look vastly different to those of a 40-year-old. It's okay to accept change, we couldn't grow as individuals without change. It's the unwillingness to adapt that sees us struggle when we should be overcoming.

There will be a difference between your priorities now and the priorities of your future self and that's the whole point of this life plan exercise. You know where you are now and where you want to be but it's getting there that is the difficult part.

Every person is unique and individual and so we don't all apply the same levels of importance to something. The list provided here is to give you an idea of what might be important and then to use them for yourself or others.

A life plan usually consists of between five to ten main priorities but I've listed more for you here as a guide to use. These are in

alphabetical order because I wouldn't want you to think that one is more important than another. For example, family might not be a priority for some people who do not get on with their family, are estranged from them, or have lost family members.

- Career.
- Children.
- Community.
- Education.
- Experiences.
- Faith.
- Family.
- Finances.
- Friendships.
- Happiness.
- Hobby.
- Mental health.
- Personal growth.
- Physical health.
- Relationships.
- Security.
- Spiritual health.
- Travel.

Having priorities written down means that you can focus on them when you feel yourself being overcome with negative emotions or thoughts. It can make the difference of getting you back on the right track or being lost on the journey of life.

Once you have your five to ten main priorities in life written down then it's time to create your goals.

Step 3: Create Goals

Goals are hugely different from priorities and it is where some people go wrong when developing a life plan. Goals are what you strive towards in the same way as reaching for a dream or aim. They help keep us focused on what we wish to achieve in life.

Priorities are the elements that you need in order to achieve those goals. For example, say your biggest priority is family then your goals could be to dedicate more time to family or plan a family trip once a year.

To make this easier for you, because that's what this book is about, I've compiled a list of the priorities used above along with possible goals you could create from each one.

Remember that you only need five to ten main priorities, anymore and you'll find yourself being distracted by which priority to fall back on.

The following pages contain guides of which goals can be created from each priority listed in the previous section.

Career

- Improving your networking skills.
- Switching careers.
- Starting your own business.
- Getting a promotion.
- Becoming an expert in your field.
- Assuming a leadership position.

Children

- To have children.
- Develop your child's social skills.
- Become aware of other's feelings.
- Spend more time with your children.
- Work on a project together.

Community

- Create a strong community group.
- Improve community relations.

- Take part in local groups.
- Set up a local group.
- Spend time with like-minded people.

Education

- Earn a certificate or qualification.
- Go to University.
- Define area of interest or skills.
- Gain more knowledge.
- Learn new skills.

Experiences

- Go on an adventure.
- Take the trip you've always wanted to take.
- Make a memorable experience with friends.
- Do something that scares you.
- Go skydiving.

Spiritual

- Attend your church more often.
- Start a blog about your faith.

- Study the history of religion.
- Become part of a faith community.
- Make regular donations to your local church.

Family

- Spend more time with family.
- Volunteer together.
- Plan a regular family meet-up.
- Organise a monthly family trip.
- Show forgiveness and gratitude more often.
- Run a movie or game night once a week.

Finances

- Pay off debt.
- Save for the future or a rainy day.
- Save for a holiday.
- Start a business.
- To feel financially secure.

Friendships

- Move on from toxic friendships.
- Be happy with friends.

- Spend more time with friends.
- Plan a friends holiday every year.
- Join a community group or club together.

Happiness

- Get involved in a fun hobby like hiking.
- Do something you enjoy on a regular basis.
- Take a mental health day once a month.
- Meet with people who make you happy on a regular basis.
- Learn to relax using meditation or mindfulness.

Hobby

- Become an expert in your hobby field.
- Take up something you believe is impossible for you.
- Read more physical books.
- Join a dance or fitness class.
- Start writing a blog or a novel.

Mental health

- Maintain your mental health disorder.
- Share your own experiences to raise awareness.
- Become more self-compassionate.
- Increase self-esteem or confidence.
- A more positive body image.

Personal growth

- Gain more confidence.
- Get along with others and yourself.
- Wake up earlier to make the most of the day.
- Let go of the past.
- Become more proactive in your own life.
- Manage stress more effectively.

Physical health

- Take regular exercise.
- Eat more plant-based foods.
- Join a sports or fitness club.
- Eat more healthily.
- Stop smoking or drinking alcohol.

Relationships

- Settling down with your soulmate.
- Actively doing things for one another.
- Be romantic whenever you can.
- Travelling or going on an adventure together.
- Be kind always.

Security

- Become financially secure.
- Secure in a relationship.
- Own a home.
- Overcome self-doubt.
- Thinking positively to overcome negativity.

Travel

- Put down the map and get lost.
- Go on an adventure.
- Take a backpacking trip.
- Go on a cruise.
- Visit a country you've always wanted to visit.

Within the goals listed above there are different time-frames that can be implemented. For example, you can set one of the following:

- Daily goal.
- Weekly goal.
- Monthly goal.
- Yearly goal.
- Lifetime goal.

A lifetime goal could be something like owning a house or settling down with your soulmate. A daily goal could be to eat more healthily or managing stress more effectively.

Step 4: Write Your Life Plan

Writing your life plan is like building a roadmap from the present to the future. You've already asked yourself the right questions for your present and future self. Now it's about getting from the present to the future.

This could be the easiest or hardest step of the life plan. It's best written on a Google document, Word document or OpenOffice document, then you can print it off and keep it somewhere safe to refer to.

If you want to do a rough roadmap to begin with then simply use a sheet of paper and pen. You never know, you might find yourself to be a creative genius, if you're not already. Your life plan can be short or long and you can put as much or as little into it as you see fit.

To help with this, there are examples of a life plan in the next section.

Here's the simplest way to put together a life plan.

- Choose between FIVE or TEN priorities.
- Create at least ONE goal for each priority.
- Write down your PRESENT feelings or situation with regards to your chosen priorities.
- Write down where you want to be in the FUTURE regarding your chosen priorities.
- Add what you need TO DO to ensure that you are on the right path to meeting your goals.

Once you've decided what is important to you in your life (priorities) then add the goals you want to achieve underneath each priority.

Below that, write down where you are at the present. This would be a combination of the answers from Step 1 and your current situation.

It's important to write down your present situation because you need to know where you're at right now.

Once you've got your priorities, goals and present written down then use the future answers from Step 1 to learn where you want to be in the future.

Action plans

To get from the present to the future, you need to have something in-between otherwise you wouldn't know how to get from point A to point B. This is where the roadmap comes in and the actions needed to take you on the journey

Example 1

If you currently struggle to get on with family but in the future want to have a good relationship with them then the following steps might be needed to achieve your goals.

Action Plan Steps

- Find time to see family more often.
- Arrange a visit once a week.
- Learn forgiveness and gratitude.
- Nurture understanding for others.

- Aim to have fun with family.
- Be more open with family members about feelings.

Example 2

If you are in debt and find it difficult to cope financially but you want to be financially secure in the future then the following steps could be included to help you achieve your goals.

Action Plan Steps

- Seek help with my debt.
- Find the right savings account.
- Put at least £2 into my savings account every week.
- Stop spending money on things I end up throwing away.
- Stop wasting money on takeaways or alcohol.
- Create a financial calendar to watch my savings rise.

Your goals and action plan should be quantifiable so that you can see a difference in what you are doing. For example, if you're putting £2 into a bank account every week then at week four you will have £8. In 50 weeks, you'll have £100. It's quantifiable because you can measure or see a change.

Another example would be if you were arranging a visit once a week to see family. You can measure it by actually turning up once a week. Remember that your life plan is adaptable so if you forgot to show up or didn't feel like it one week then you can catch up the next week.

Want to move to fortnightly visits? That's fine too, as long you are making progression towards your future goals. You could even draw up a table or use the calendar on your phone to mark when you have been to visit and when you haven't. It might also be an idea to note down why you didn't do it and then look deeper into the reasons why and see what might need to change within the life plan.

It's also important to review your plan weekly, monthly or at other regular intervals to ensure that you are on track towards your goals, dreams and desired life.

Life Plan Example

To use your life plan, all you have to do is check it on a regular basis to see if you're on track or to make any changes. If you feel yourself worrying about your priorities or feeling like you're going astray then you can look at your life plan and see what you should be doing to stay on the right path.

This life plan example contains two priorities whereas yours should include at least five. As this is only an example, I haven't filled out the book with them.

You can use this example as a template, guide, or marker to help you write your own. Some people create more visual style life plans in the form of tables, graphs, or slide shows. Whatever works for you is the right way to do it.

My Suicide Prevention Life Plan (Example)

I'm writing my life plan to ensure my future is a positive one full of love and joy. At the time of writing I'm mostly a negative person who doesn't get on with my family and is in financial debt. I'm creating my life plan to help me change that.

Through self-questioning both my present and future self I've discovered what is important in my life and have created goals around them.

Family

I aim to have a happy and fruitful relationship with my family members. To help achieve this I will find time to see my family more often and arrange a visit once a week. During each visit, I want to do something special with my family such as a game night, a nice meal or quality time to talk.

My goal is to have fun with my family and nurture understanding and love for one another. I aim to show forgiveness and gratitude freely and be more open with family members about my feelings.

Finances

My goal is to be financially secure, having saved for the future. To reach my goal I'm going to seek help with my debt and then find the right savings account to use. I will aim to save a minimum of £2.00 per week.

To help in my goals I will stop spending money on things I end up throwing away. I will also stop wasting money on takeaways and alcohol and instead aim to save the money in my new savings account. I will create a financial calendar so I can see my savings increase on a regular basis.

In your life plan, you can even include the answers to some of the questions you asked yourself in the future as a marker for where you want to be. Generally, life plans are written in paragraphs as above but you can be more visual if it works for you.

There's no right or wrong way to create a life plan. Enjoy it, use it and you could reap the benefits.

Organisations & Helplines

UNITED KINGDOM

MIND

Mental health charity that offers information and advice to people with mental health problems and lobbies government and local authorities on their behalf. It also works to raise public awareness and understanding of issues relating to mental health. Founded in 1946.

www.mind.org.uk

SAMARITANS

Samaritans is a registered charity aimed at providing emotional support to anyone in emotional distress, struggling to cope, or at risk of suicide throughout the United Kingdom and Ireland, often through their telephone helpline.

www.samaritans.org or call: **116 123**

RETHINK MENTAL ILLNESS

Mental health charity helping people severely affected by mental illness to improve their lives. They are on a mission to bring about meaningful change through services, groups and ground-breaking campaigns.

www.rethink.org

SANE

SANE is a leading UK mental health charity working to improve quality of life for people affected by mental illness.

www.sane.org.uk or call: **0300 304 7000**

CALM

CALM (Campaign Against Living Miserably) is a free, confidential and anonymous helpline as well as a webchat service, offering help, advice and information to anyone who is struggling or in crisis.

www.thecalmzone.net or call: **0800 58 58 58**

HOPELINE UK

PAPYRUS is the national charity dedicated to the prevention of young suicide. They provide a helpline for those under 35-years-old experiencing thoughts of suicide.

www.papyrus-uk.org/hopelineuk or call: **0800 068 41 41**

SHOUT

The UK's first free 24/7 text service for anyone in crisis anytime, anywhere. It is a place to go for those struggling to cope and in need of immediate help

www.giveusashout.org or text **HELP** to **85258**

UNITED STATES

LIFELINE

National suicide prevention helpline. The Lifeline provides 24/7, free and confidential support for people in distress, prevention and crisis resources for you or your loved ones, and best practices for professionals.

www.suicidepreventionlifeline.org or call **1-800-273-8255**

THE TREVOR PROJECT

The Trevor Project is the leading national organization providing crisis intervention and suicide prevention services to lesbian, gay, bisexual, transgender and queer (LGBTQ) young people under 25.

www.thetrevorproject.org or call: **1-866-488-7386**

DIDI HIRSCH SUICIDE PREVENTION CENTER

Didi Hirsch's Suicide Prevention Center helps over 100,000 people a year, saving lives throughout the nation and world. They offer crisis services, therapy, support, training and also participate in leading edge research that is transforming the field and saving lives.

www.didihirsch.org or call: **800-273-8255.**

2-1-1

2-1-1 is an essential resource helpline for overcoming personal barriers and challenges. Their trained professionals connect you with the relevant local resource in your State or County.

www.211.org or call: **211**

ANY OTHER COUNTRY

BEFRIENDERS WORLDWIDE

Befrienders Worldwide is a charity that connects to 349 emotional support centres in 32 countries, spanning 5 continents. These centres are staffed by more than 25,000 volunteers who provide vital support to an estimated 7 million service users each year.

Select your country to find your relevant helplines.

www.befrienders.org

List of UK Resources

I hope you find this list of sites helpful. All links have been checked for recent activity, quality, and relevancy, as of Summer 2021.

Action For Happiness – www.actionforhappiness.org

Alzheimer's Research UK – www.alzheimersresearchuk.org

Alzheimer's Society – www.alzheimers.org.uk

Anxiety UK – www.anxietyuk.org.uk

Aware – www.aware-ni.org

Big White Wall – www.bigwhitewall.com

Bipolar UK – www.bipolaruk.org

Breathing Space – www.breathingspace.scot

Carers UK – www.carersuk.org

Centre For Mental Health – www.centreformentalhealth.org.uk

Childline – www.childline.org.uk

Citizens Advice – www.citizensadvice.org.uk

Combat Stress – www.combatstress.org.uk

Doctor's Support Network – www.dsn.org.uk

Get Connected – www.getconnected.org.uk

Heads Together – www.headstogether.org.uk

Hearing Voices Network – www.hearing-voices.org

Inter Voice – www.intervoiceonline.org

Kooth – www.kooth.com

LGBT Switchboard – www.switchboard.lgbt

Lifesigns – www.lifesigns.org.uk

Maytree – www.maytree.org.uk

Mental Health Foundation – www.mentalhealth.org.uk

Mental Health UK – www.mentalhealth-uk.org

MindEd – www.mindedforfamilies.org.uk

Moodscope – www.moodscope.com

Muslim Youth Helpline – www.myh.org.uk

National Self Harm Network – www.nshn.co.uk

Nightline – www.nightline.ac.uk

OCD Action – www.ocdaction.org.uk

OCD UK – www.ocduk.org

PANDAS Foundation – www.pandasfoundation.org.uk

Place2Be – www.place2be.org.uk

Relate – www.relate.org.uk

Safe In Our World – www.safeinourworld.org

SAMH (Scotland's Mental Health) – www.samh.org.uk

Self-Harm UK – www.selfharm.co.uk

Student Minds – www.studentminds.org.uk

Students Against Depression – www.studentsagainstdepression.org

Support Line – www.supportline.org.uk

The Mix – www.themix.org.uk

Time To Change – www.time-to-change.org.uk

Together - www.together-uk.org

United Response – www.unitedresponse.org.uk

Young Minds – www.youngminds.org.uk

"We need hopes and dreams in our lives because without them, we're running on empty."

Glossary

ASD: Acute stress disorder.

AMHP: Approved Mental Health Professional. A decision over sectioning is usually carried out by at least two approved mental health professionals who are normally mental health nurses or psychiatrists.

AMHT: The Acute Mental Health Team provide intensive support for people who are experiencing an acute, or a 'crisis' episode during their mental illness.

BDD: Body dysmorphic disorder.

BPD: Borderline personality disorder.

CMHT: The Community Mental Health Team. They provide non-intensive mental health care in and around the community.

DENP: An acronym for the levels of urgency in a conversation. Stands for Dangerous, Emotional, Negative and Positive.

DID: Dissociative identity disorder

DISCONNECT: A feeling of not being in reality at any given moment.

DRAINING: The consequential physical effect of mentally overworking the brain.

EUPD: Emotionally unstable personality disorder, which is another term for BPD.

EXIGENT PHASE: A time during a mental health crisis when urgent help is necessary.

GAD: General Anxiety Disorder.

GROUNDING: The skill of bringing yourself back in to the present moment using various grounding techniques.

IMMORTAL HOUR: Mentally trapped in a moment of time that comes to define a person.

MENTACRACY: The rule of mental illness over a person's everyday life.

MENTAL HEALTH ACT: The Mental Health Act 1983, is an Act of the Parliament of the United Kingdom which applies to people in England and Wales. It covers the reception, care and treatment of mentally disordered persons, the management of their property and other related matters.

MENTAL ILLNESS: A mental health problem that significantly affects how a person feels, thinks, behaves, and interacts with other people. There are many types of mental illness such as mood disorders, personality disorders and psychotic disorders.

MINDFULNESS: The quality or state of being conscious or aware of something in the present moment. It means to ground yourself and your thoughts in the present.

NSSI: Non-suicidal self-injury.

PMR: Progressive Muscle Relaxation. The method of tensing and relaxing muscles to relieve stress and tension.

PTSD: Post Traumatic Stress Disorder.

SKYLINED: The belief that upon death, a human soul becomes a star.

SUICIDE PREVENTION LIFE PLAN: A roadmap for your life that helps you find what is important to you and helps focus your attention on moving towards your desired life.

TELEOLOGY: The philosophical explanation of phenomena in terms of the purpose they serve rather than of the cause by which they arise.

WITHDRAWAL: The physical and mental process of removing oneself from the real world.

Bibliography

Selected bibliography with references and suggested reading.

Advani S, Kochhar G, Chachra S, Dhawan P. *Eating everything except food (PICA): A rare case report and review.* J Int Soc Prev Community Dent. 2014;4(1):1-4.

Barker, Clive. *Sacrament.* HarperCollins, 1996.

Bible Society. *Belief in angels poll.* https://www.biblesociety.org.uk/latest/news/a-third-of-all-brits-believe-in-guardian-angels, 2016.

British Government website page on how to get help if you feel you are suffering or know someone who is suffering from domestic abuse https://www.gov.uk/guidance/domestic-abuse-how-to-get-help

Demyttenaere, K., Bruffaerts, R., Posada-Villa, J., Gasquet, I., Kovess, V., Lepine, J.P., ... & Chatterji, S. *Prevalence, severity, and unmet need for treatment of mental disorders in the World Health Organization.* World Mental Health Surveys. JAMA, 292(21), 2581–2590, 2004.

Gutman, Joshi, Parsonage & Schoon. *Children of the New Century. Millennium Cohort Study,* 2015 (with data collected in 2012).

Hawthorne, Nathaniel. *The Scarlet Letter.* Ticknor, Reed & Fields, 1850.

Hipparchus. *Precession of the Equinoxes,* Britannica, July 1998. https://www.britannica.com/science/precession-of-the-equinoxes

HM Government. *Carers at the heart of the 21stcentury families and communities.* London: Department of Health. Sourced from gov.uk/government/publications/the-national-carers-strategy , 2008.

International Telecommunications Union. Global ITC Developments. 2018.

Johnson, Monte Ransome. *Aristotle on Teleology*, Clarendon, 2005.

Keel PK, Klump KL. *Are eating disorders culture-bound syndromes?* Implications for conceptualizing their etiology. Psychol Bull. 2003;129(5):747-769.

Mitchell, David. *Cloud Atlas.* Hodder & Stoughton. ISBN: 9780340822784

NHS Digital. Spreadsheets on self-harm, suicide and hospital visits. https://digital.nhs.uk

Oakley, Ben. Mentacracy: Living Under The Rule Of Mental Illness. ISBN: 9781707499410

ONS (Office for National Statistics) *Suicides in the United Kingdom: 2017 Registrations.* Retrieved from: https://www.ons.gov.uk/peoplepopulationandcommunit... 4th Sept 2018.

Sempik, J., & Becker, S. Young Adult Carers at School Experiences and Perceptions of Caring and Education. Carers Trust. 2013.

Shah, A.J., Wadoo, O., & Latoo, J. *Review Article: Psychological Distress in Carers of People with Mental Disorders.* British Journal of Medical Practitioners, 3(3), 327. 2010.

St Germain SA, Hooley JM. Direct and indirect forms of non-suicidal self-injury: evidence for a distinction. Psychiatry Res. 2012;197(1-2):78-84.

Thompson, Hunter. S. *Fear & Loathing in Las Vegas.* HarperCollins Publishers. ISBN: 9780007204496

World Health Organization (WHO) – *SUPRE: Suicide Prevention.* https://www.who.int/mental_health/prevention/suicide/supresuicideprevent/en

Acknowledgements

Our individual guardian angels.

Every mental health worker in public and private practices, you are needed more than you know.

All the mental health charities working tirelessly to give people a better life.

To the effort that goes into maintaining statistics so that we may better understand the extent of mental health. And thank you to those who care.

To the sufferers and families of those who are in pain or no longer with us.

You are not alone and you are loved.

For more books, research, and articles, visit:

www.benoakley.co.uk

Printed in Great Britain
by Amazon

82088150R00122